"This book is a must-read for any yoga practitioner or teacher who wants to dive deeper into the understanding of yoga—mind, body, and spirit."
—SUZANNE MCCAHILL PERRINE, yoga teacher and Ayurveda Health Coach

"Mary's singular, humble voice rises above the clamor and ushers us into a new way of learning and being, where curiosity is paramount and one's own unique, direct experience is the ultimate authority. A must-read for all aspiring yogis."
—MELISSA SHALONGO, yoga teacher

Teach People,
Not Poses

LESSONS IN YOGA ANATOMY AND
FUNCTIONAL MOVEMENT TO
UNLOCK BODY INTELLIGENCE

Mary Richards, MS

WITH ILLUSTRATIONS BY LILI ROBINS

FOREWORD BY JUDITH HANSON LASATER, PHD, PT

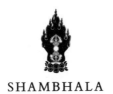

SHAMBHALA

Shambhala Publications, Inc.
2129 13th Street
Boulder, Colorado 80302
www.shambhala.com

Cover art: ace03/shutterstock
Cover design: Katrina Noble
Interior design: Katrina Noble

9 8 7 6 5 4 3 2 1

First Edition
Printed in the United States of America

Shambhala Publications makes every effort to print on acid-free, recycled paper.
Shambhala Publications is distributed worldwide by Penguin Random
House, Inc., and its subsidiaries.

LIBRARY OF CONGRESS CATALOGING-IN-PUBLICATION DATA
Names: Richards, Mary (Yoga teacher), author. | Robins, Lili, illustrator.
    | Lasater, Judith, author of foreword.
Title: Teach people, not poses: lessons in yoga anatomy and functional
    movement to unlock body intelligence / Mary Richards, M.S.; with
    illustrations by Lili Robins; foreword by Judith Hanson Lasater, Ph.D., P.T.
Description: Boulder, Colorado: Shambhala, [2023]
Identifiers: LCCN 2022056340 | ISBN 9781611809725 (trade paperback)
Subjects: LCSH: Yoga—Study and teaching.
Classification: LCC RA781.67 .R53 2023 | DDC 613.7/046071—dc23/eng/20221223
LC record available at https://lccn.loc.gov/2022056340

CONTENTS

FOREWORD

Rarely in life do we come upon a book that makes us exclaim, "I am so happy someone finally wrote this book." *Teach People, Not Poses* is such a book.

Notably this book is not just another book about asana practice. Rather, it is a sourcebook for personal practice and for learning the scientific basis of how and why yoga works. It carefully leads the reader through the logical and specific processes that define movement principles. This helps us not just to understand those principles but also to begin *to embody them.*

An outstanding theme of the book is the emphasis Mary Richards places on the individual nature of practice. Often in yoga classes, students are all told to do the exact same thing and to continue to repeat the same poses in the same way every week. But *Teach People, Not Poses* is true to its title and continually reinforces that to practice yoga is to become intimate with our own body—its strengths, weaknesses, and challenges—and then to explore the poses from a foundation of this self-knowledge.

One of my favorite passages is: (This book) "is an offering of science-based information and skill-building activities to equip you for your very own asana expeditions as well as support your teaching, if you lead others in yoga movement." Mary teaches us by empowering us to look inward, to trust our own bodies and our own experience, and to proceed with curiosity and confidence.

Another favorite quote is "An essential truth of practice is that there is no yoga without you." I would add that there is no sophisticated, knowledgeable, and effective yoga practice without the deep and useful information that Mary shares with us in this book.

I cannot recommend this book more highly. I predict it will become a classic for yoga students and teachers alike. So read this book, slowly and carefully. Practice what it offers and savor it for its depth, honesty, and usefulness. I have no doubt that you will be delighted with the result.

Judith Hanson Lasater, PhD, PT

Teach People,
Not Poses

INTRODUCTION

Teach People, Not Poses encapsulates some of the path-shaping influences that have guided my personal yoga practice and teaching over the last thirty years. It's meant as a guidebook, to help everyone build a robust foundation for the many aspects of practice. My focus centers around ideas and strategies to release the form of each asana from within the individual person, rather than conforming the person to preconceived "display rules" of the pose. We all know square pegs don't fit in round holes, and this book is an attempt at helping everyone sort through such mismatches. In other words, teach people, not poses.

After all, the entire purpose of asana practice is to go spelunking into the deeply personal and intimate spaces of the body. It's a journey into the pulsating, vibrating energies and feelings flowing between and within the cells and, thus, the psyche. By yoking the attention with the multitude of fluctuations living through our tissues, asana helps us connect to the essential wisdom that the only constancy in life is change. Not only is every Triangle Pose (Trikonasana) the first time you are practicing *that* Triangle Pose, but this is also true for everyone else—new or experienced practitioner, teacher, or student. The beautiful reality is that everybody is unique, just like everyone else. Since every asana is unique, too, its practice provides an infinitely rich context to learn more about our bodies and ourselves.

To be fair, one of my many biases is that yoga practice begins and lives with the body through its many states. This is my way of saying that this book is by no means, no how a complete exposition of yoga or its practice. Though my practice began on the philosophical side with the Bhagavad Gita, it wasn't until I began asana and pranayama practice at age twenty-two, in 1992, that I felt the integrative effects of yoga. I personally couldn't fathom, much less embody, the heart-opening, mind-soothing, and soul-liberating residues of the Gita without starting in my flesh and bone. So I picked up a copy of B. K. S. Iyengar's *Light on Yoga*, unrolled a sticky mat, and have not rolled it up since—except to move it around.

At the beginning, my practice was largely self-taught. As I mentioned, the first asana book I purchased all those years ago was Iyengar's *Light on Yoga*. My bookshelves have long been packed with yoga books, many chock-full of photographs of lovely people displaying spectacular asana. And through no fault but my own, I spent decades chasing those images because I had conflated the picture with the "real" asana in myself and others.

I believe it is hugely important to see images of a wide diversity of folks doing anything and everything. We have long delayed the undeniable and righteous imperatives of inclusivity, equity, and justice on and off the mat. However, when we look at any picture, we are looking at a captured moment in the past of another person, outside our presence. Some of us, at least, need a different sort of visual reference.

One of the reasons this book features custom illustrations called avatars in lieu of photographs is to reframe the visual narrative of asana instruction. The avatars germinated from my own iPencil-drawn stick figures, which I've long used as a teaching tool in dozens of workshops and online courses. So, I came up with an idea for using hand-drawn avatars that could serve as "blanks." The forty-five figures created by my illustrator, Lili Robins, attempt to clear the observational clutter that arises when trying to see yourself or others in images that don't line up with what your eyes behold in real time.

The avatars are intended as flexible, every-person representations, to spare both the square peg and the round hole.

The illustrations also serve as an homage to a few of my favorite, formative yoga and movement books. Blandine Calais-Germain, Moshe Feldenkrais, and others relied on posable art mannequins and line drawings to communicate the essence of their anatomy and movement lessons. The neutrality and creative intimacy of their book art helped open my view to the subtle and individual. By leaving more to the imagination, the illustrations allowed me to recognize and fill in the details from my own observational and felt experience. It is my intention that the avatars in this book offer similar opportunities for you, dear reader. Think of them as customizable Memojis.

The primary focus of *Teach People, Not Poses* is directed at building practical body knowledge and physical core stabilization skills to engage in enjoyable individualized asana. To promote synergistic benefits, the strength and motion control training is combined with the salubrious effects of pranayama and contemplative rest. While informed by accredited education in body and yoga science, every lesson included here is derived from my experiences with thousands of students. The information and exercises leverage time and effort for functional gains that minimize risk and encourage safety in asana and beyond. Chapter 1 sheds some light on where I'm coming from.

There's anatomy talk, but only as it pertains to developing fluency in how we are put together and how structure dictates the direction and range of movement available to any given person. In discussing body structure, the emphasis is on seeing the person in the mirror of your gaze and recognizing widely encountered anatomical and postural configurations. Specifically, the body mapping and alignment grid activities—in Chapters 2 and 3, respectively—help us see how a person's bones and joints are stacked and connected in Mountain Pose (Tadasana). When we can identify the structural and postural idiosyncrasies of the person standing in front of us, we are able to follow and guide their anatomical forms into asana shapes that arise naturally from within the individual. This is a key skill in asana and life: the ability to see and recognize the living person in front of us. It's harder than we think but worth the difficulty for the ease and contentment that flow from lifting the veil.

In addition to anatomy, there are several lessons in kinesiology, or the science of movement. No discussion of anatomy and asana, no matter how brief, is complete without framing the conversation in the context of movement in a sea of gravity. Seriously, if you aren't obsessed with gravity yet, what are you waiting for?! It comes to bear in all movement in every single person on earth, whether bendy as a willow or stiff as a board. Gravity is so important to our movement that we even have a gyroscope of sorts in our bodies, located right above the bladder—yes, the sac that holds urine. Since the gravitational center is located in the deep belly, Chapter 4 is an expedition into the form, function, and intersection of forces in the pelvis—the seat of all movement. Indeed, the ability to tune in and stay connected to the gravitational center of the body is widely accepted and promulgated by movement-centric, behavioral, and psychological therapists alike as an essential skill to nourish overall health and well-being.

Some of the concepts and descriptions of various structures, systems, and functions can get a little Nerdy Wordy, so there are tables to break things down—and build them up—from the familiar to the technical. You will see these informational and linguistic turnouts in Chapters 2, 3, and 4. Please prioritize patience and gentleness when parsing through the Greek and Latin, both literally and figuratively. More important than memorizing terms or reciting cues is to stop, see, and smell the roses of simply being present. There is plenty of time to get more comfortable with the body, to learn more about its contours, cadences, and challenges. The asana abides within us, so it's inevitable that the eyes, brain, and body come together.

In fact, the more consciously and deliberately we move, the easier it becomes for brain and body, body and brain to come together. Slow and steady wins the proverbial race. That said, the fastest route to feeling centered, stable, and at ease—yet ready to move—is by way of the belly. The roundhouse of neuromusculoskeletal stabilization and motion control systems located within and around the trunk is where most of the integrative magic happens. Thus, Chapters 5 and 6 are dedicated to daily physical training exercises, to develop strong, responsive tissues and patterning intuition to get organized for more complex or higher amplitude asana. To move safely and efficiently, stability comes first. That's just the way of it. It's literally why we have so many checks and balances and built-in redundancies in our anatomy, physiology, and neurology. Check out the tables that detail the gazillion muscles and fascial structures of the body's stabilization systems. The sheer magnitude of tissue offers ample evidence of stability's primacy in our ability to get up, down, and all around.

Physical conditioning requires consistency. Quantity of practice does help move things along. In a perfect world, we should practice each core training series in its entirety on alternating days or every day in tandem once the body can carry the load without resentment. That means no rushing; no overworking; no overburdening the body, breath, and/or mind. It's far healthier and more productive to do an exercise or two per day than not to do anything at all because you cannot do the entire series for whatever reason. Start with one exercise and one round of breath. Do that one pose for one cycle of breath. That's how change starts and starting lines change: with one breath and one movement yoked together by attentiveness.

Asana helps us cultivate capacities for the attention, concentration, courage, stamina, strength, and tenderness needed to connect fully to beingness. It does not work alone nor is it meant to, however well-intentioned and skillfully executed. Whether seeking to influence movement progression or stress reactivity, asana with pranayama and meditative rest form a triumvirate of practices that nurtures beneficial changes in physical, mental, emotional, and spiritual resilience and responsiveness. Chapter 7, therefore, outlines some of the whys and how-tos of specific breathing exercises and restorative asana. Furthermore, most of us are tired—exhausted, even. At the very least, our tissues need a breather, especially when challenged to learn new things or to recover and repair from fatigue and injury. Quiet practices offer another potent benefit: in learning how and when to apply restorative yoga techniques, practitioners can learn to reframe their relationship with pain and dysfunction and cultivate conditions that enliven feelings of safety and contentment. Chapter 8 includes some closing thoughts about the upside of becoming more welcoming to ourselves.

I began teaching asana and pranayama classes in 2000 by accident. I was pregnant with the first of my two children, working full-time, and I had zero aspirations to lead others in practice. However, one of my teachers at the time saw something in me. After class one evening, she flat-out told me that I would begin teaching as an apprentice in her home-based studio, under her supervision, the very next week. For some reason, I said yes.

Fast-forward to today and I am still saying yes—and getting more excited about my practice and teaching as time goes on. The world and life become so much bigger, yet more intimate at the same time. The more I learn, the less I know. The less I know, the more curious I feel. The more curious I feel, the more connected to Self I become. I take all this to mean that home lives inside us wherever we find ourselves—and when we feel at home inside, we are connected to our agency and autonomy. The feeling of empowerment fed by curiosity-enabled connection is the sole dominion of the individual. While no one can take it away, our sense of self and safety networks get scrambled or interrupted at times.

Challenging circumstances may seem to cut us off from feeling centered, safe, and free. Pain, suffering, and separation from the grounded center of being might even feel insurmountable. I have looked at the road of life ahead and felt the dread of navigating its course. Yet every time I have needed to adjust my bearings to find clarity and contentment, the exact resources have revealed themselves and helped me make it back home to myself. From books to people who reflect my shadows and radiance, I am living proof that the universe looks after fools and innocents.

This book, in fact, was ultimately born from one such crossing of paths a couple decades ago. After a pair of rotator cuff and sacroiliac joint injuries that occurred with the instructor du jour's hands on me, I became a question-asking nuisance in asana classes, trainings, and workshops. So much so that one of my regular asana teachers, in a fit of pique, told me to go see Judith Hanson Lasater if I was going to persist in my burgeoning love affair with anatomy and kinesiology in asana. I was raised to put my money where my mouth is, so when this teacher told me to seek out Judith, that is exactly what I did.

In September 2002, I registered for a weekend workshop with Judith dedicated to the shoulder in Charlottesville, Virginia. Over the course of the weekend, Judith helped me find my pelvis and restore the natural congruence of my sacroiliac joints in Mountain and Triangle Poses. (Yes, in my experience, you can lose track of your pelvis. See Chapter 4.) She also helped me eliminate the nagging pain in my right shoulder, which had persisted for well over a year despite graduating from physical therapy and receiving a cortisone injection. Per Judith's intervention in Downward-Facing Dog Pose (Adho Mukha Svanasana) that weekend, I haven't had a problem in this pose since. My heart has also grown at least 108 times larger since that weekend because of the wildly engaging sisterhood that I share with Judith to this day.

Teach People, Not Poses is thus inspired, in substance and title, by the words of my dear friend, mentor, and teacher: "As yoga teachers, we teach people, not poses." These words have been my mantra for many years. Taking a person-centric approach to asana instruction has saved a lot of grief and effort on the mat, both for me and for my students. Rather than striving to actualize idealized forms made popular by various lineages and commercial outlets, let's allow our bodies to lead our asana practice. The body is going to have the final say in what's sustainable anyhow. We might as well surrender and follow where our individual anatomy and strain tolerances allow us to move.

I owe a profound debt of gratitude to every student whose mat I have darkened with my looming presence, probing eyes, and surprisingly powerful finger-pointing skills. My students taught me to surrender my ideas and beliefs about width of base and shoulder positions. They showed me where rotation, flexion, extension, and other movements really come from in their bodies—and the many ways folks fake it or take risks to make it. In sum, my students taught me to see them as people, not poses. For them, for my mentor, for my colleagues, I share this collection of lessons in honor of the inestimable privilege afforded to me as a yoga teacher and human. May this guidebook further enable you to practice and live in harmony with your body, breath, mind, heart, and spirit.

1

Yoga Curious

WHERE PRACTICE BEGINS

Blessed are the curious, for they shall have adventures.
—Lovelle Drachman[1]

Each of us meets yoga in our own way, yet many of us tread a common path into the world of practice. We frequently begin our journey by stepping onto the mat for physical training through asana. Some of us undertake pose practice to explore a different type of movement. Others seek relief from chronic pain, strain, and stress. Still others search for metaphysical understanding. Whatever the motivation or intention, asana invites the yoga-curious individual on a quest of self-study that begins with the body.

Asana offers a reliable route to learn more about how, when, and where we feel sensations. Since poses originate from archetypal shapes and organic energies that exist within us, they also help us trace connections between our bodily sensations and our feelings, thoughts, and beliefs. Practice is a kind of personal anthropology, delving into the realities and relationships between soma, soul, self, and society. Any given asana invites us to explore along spectrums of form and function, ease and exertion, attitude and behavior—from outright rebellion to peaceful acceptance, or at least bemused resignation. We are, in essence, navigating pathways on a somato-sensory map toward a pin labeled "Mountain Pose."

When we first start looking for Mountain Poses in our bodies, we typically benefit from well-tried approaches to the mountaintop. A trustworthy itinerary crafted by an experienced voyager offers a credible way to prioritize time, effort, and other resources. Inspired by the findings and wisdom shared by those who have made the trip before us, we are emboldened to open up to new places, practices, and perspectives.

As we grow more familiar with ourselves on the mat, however, it behooves us to undertake asana via more personalized pathways. After all, the necessity for a metaphorical change of scenery may be what brought us to the mat in the first place. To deepen and expand our self-study, we must blaze trails for ourselves in harmony with our individual conformation and psyche. Otherwise, our physical and spiritual inquiries become ensnared in closed loops of tradition, where our desire for self-knowing is compressed by inherent tendencies toward doctrinal correctness.

Off the Beaten Path: Become Your Own Guide

No matter the consistency or longevity of our practice, asana entails the unity of attention and intention with the spirit of openhearted-ness. It also calls for a willingness to step out of line and examine the status quo while trusting the embodied wisdom of our own gut instincts and felt senses. Trust, however, can prove to be a sticky wicket.

Many of us question our self-worth and sagacity. We may not be able to articulate the source of our doubts for a wealth of reasons. Yet hankerings toward some sort of reorientation in perspective, effort, or objective tend to make their presence felt. We might even hear a voice inside or see an inner vision beckoning us further into ourselves. We intuit where the rubber meets the road in how we respond to changes of heart, direction, or mind.

A headlong rush into the wilderness is certainly one way to get out of our comfort zone. On the other hand, we may choose to rein in, or even prevent, any sort of wanderlust from taking hold. Sometimes our preferences for predictability and comity encourage us to cling to authority figures and their ideas long after we have outgrown the need to follow in another's footsteps.

Whatever your go-to strategies for self-examination, keep in mind that asana instruction is tradition-dominant and rules-based. Its ingrained tendency is toward compliance and consistency. Principles about hows and shoulds organize methods for practice: how bones should stack to create pose shapes, how to adjust internal pressures and the benefits of doing so, and how to direct the vital energies to nourish well-being and inner peace. The reasoning behind the rules is enmeshed in an intricate web of sociocultural forces, with the profusion of threads cast toward younger bodies residing on the male end of the gender spectrum. Instructions such as "square the pelvis," "glue your sitting bones to the floor," and "engage Mula Bandha" can work well enough for prepubescent bodies but wreak havoc with more mature bodies. Bodies with any sort of gynecological history are not well served by many espoused cues. By "gynecological history," I mean menstruation, hormone therapies, fertility and pregnancy experiences, surgical or vaginal childbirth, and so on.

Sooner or later, in that one pesky pose or perhaps several, the status quo of popularized asana instruction loses its luster in the context of the individual. Points of departure come, regardless of biology, whenever our autonomy catches up with our sensitivity and awareness. Sometimes our self-reliance is helped along by acute injury, chronic conditions, or seismic life events. Multiply changes in physicality and emotionality by the weight of the day-to-day, and we have an equation for recalibration. We usually determine that we must adapt our practice to grow and thrive—on and off the mat.

As our sense of the world widens, the impetus arises to unleash our curiosity, challenge conventional wisdom, and create opportunities to learn more about ourselves. We dream about roads less traveled. We consider the skills, gear, and information needed to visit new sights. We think about exploring at our own pace, according to our own inclinations. We sense the potential to build bridges with the body, mind, heart, and spirit.

Freedom to Roam: Curiosity, Consent, and Boundaries

My first divergence from the "authorized" and "certified" asana systems that structured my methods came about ten years into my practice. A shoulder injury invited me to venture into the vast unknown of how my body really worked and felt during asana. The injury was induced by a commonly applied assist during a led Ashtanga *vinyasa* class. Though I received prompt sports medicine care, it became a chronic nuisance thanks to my own strict adherence to yoga-specific instructions pertaining to arm position.

Downward-Facing Dog was especially troublesome. I felt some degree of pain every time I practiced it with the suite of commonly deployed cues: shoulder blades held firmly in the midback, pulling the inner-upper corners down toward the waist; upper arms externally rotated, forearms internally rotated; upper traps relaxed; chest toward the thighs, hollow belly; sitting bones lifted; and so on. I began to dread and loathe my practice of this pose—and I am a dog aficionado from mat to kennel. I knew something needed to change for me in the pose, even though I simultaneously believed I was surely doing something "wrong" despite my front-of-the-class, good-student fervor. Basically, misery led me into the uncharted territory of understanding my own anatomy and autonomy.

As mentioned previously, I attended a three-day workshop about the anatomy and kinesiology of the shoulder about a month out from this dustup that shifted the course of my shoulder—and my sacroiliac joints. Not only did I physically feel better thanks to what I learned in that workshop, but I took home an even bigger lesson from the weekend: curiosity is the wellspring from which communication, connection, understanding, and thus the potential for empathy and compassion flows. Courtesy and consent form the boundaries that safely channel interactions on the mat within and between practitioners and teachers. Judith was the first teacher to ask me—and listen to—how I felt in a pose. We shared a give-and-take on the mat rather than simply repeating the "this-is-how-it-is-done" rules. She was also the first teacher to explain how she would like to place props or her hands on me and sought my consent before laying a finger on my person. Asana practice and teaching upended, I realized that I needed to reflect on a whole lot more than my shoulders.

Expect the Unexpected:
Bruised Egos and Bumps in the Road

There's fluidity between authority and autonomy in the teacher-student relationship—as well as between the inner child and outward adult. Learning, after all, is a collaborative effort where we balance support and structure with challenge and independence. We tend to rely on authority and take autonomy for granted, a.k.a. "better safe than sorry." Fear of shame makes it easy to conflate familiarity with safety, curiosity with disrespect, and growth with regret. Resolution of the shoulder situation opened my eyes to these tensions on my own and others' mats.

Despite all the decades of sports and athletic training that told me otherwise, I had relentlessly adhered to asana instructions that didn't make sense or suit me. And I blamed myself for any problems that arose. My self-suppression makes sense, especially in retrospect; after all, I was practicing yoga-specific movements. Play the game, play by its rules. Furthermore, the techniques and philosophy of yoga were birthed oceans and eons away from my life. I had several centuries of ground to cover, so the guidance of fellow seekers who had more education, training, and experience benefited me immensely.

However, I had surrendered curiosity about how my body worked and felt on the mat to the authority of widely recognized "masters." I viewed every sensation from the outside in, seeking external validation because I did not trust my own wisdom and experience. I believed others knew more about how a body should feel, move, and look than I knew about my own. By abdicating my autonomy, I ended up exactly where I had begun my yoga journey more than a decade earlier: lost. So I decided to go where my feet took me and have a look around.

Perhaps it is needless to say, but I'm going to do it anyway: the workshop did not cure my preoccupation with anatomy and kinesiology. I began taking body, health, and movement science courses at local state and community colleges. I attended workshop after workshop with senior yoga teachers. I also spent a tremendous amount of time as a physical therapy (PT) patient, thanks to another commonly used assist that shredded my right hip and a hiking accident that tore up my left knee. I ate a lot of crow, tended to my bruised ego, and retired much of my asana training as I learned more in academic and therapeutic environs about the body, its variations, and movement strategies in relationship to gravity.

Uncovering ways to work around obstacles was encouraged by the students and fellow teachers who came to me on the mat. I noted correlations between frequently touted alignment cues and the musculoskeletal injuries and imbalances that I was seeing on the mat. I gathered loads of anecdotal data, especially from folks with female bodies; larger bodies; older bodies; and bodies with observable and/or documented anatomical variations, acute injuries, chronic complaints, and replacement parts. I continued to put many sacred cows of alignment out to pasture in my own teaching and practice. I noted the changes in myself and corroborated positive effects with those who came to me for instruction.

I started to see my students not as potential poses but as people who drive cars, ride bicycles, play tennis and golf, carry babies, run for miles, and go on scuba-diving vacations. I noted the functional overlays of repetitive activities as well as the residue of habitual sedentary positions that I saw in "desk drivers." I paid attention to the small movement adjustments made by students to arrange themselves into, within, and out of asana. My observations led me to question everything I had been told to do, the whys behind the telling, and how I told others to practice on the mat.

Prepare for Adventure: Yoga Ready

The initial conception of a pose arises in the prefrontal cortex at the front of the brain. Let's take Warrior II Pose (Virabhadrasana II) as an example. The vision of Warrior II forms in the mind's eye, then works its way through the network of neurons, fascial layers, and muscle units to arrange the body's bones and joints. The body's feeling of Warrior II travels from the flesh back up to the base of the brain, where the cerebellum performs a quality check. We adapt in response to feedback to ensure that we have or can acquire what we need to abide in the pose we hope to express.

The asana-finding process is best nourished by patience, fascination, regularity, and kind regard. Directed by these values, every one of us can connect to the energetic vibe of any asana we choose within the context of our individuality. To do so safely requires us to become exquisitely intimate with the features, shapes, sensations, feelings, and energies of our own bodies.

That's where this book comes into play: it is an offering of science-based information and skill-building activities to equip you for your very own asana expeditions as well as to support your teaching, if you lead others in yoga movement. It even includes some language lessons to help you find your way around the body. Think of it as a travel guide, with all sorts of recommendations to uncover hidden gems and tucked-away places that will invigorate your inner wisdom and inherent radiance.

First, we will learn to map the bony features that indicate skeletal structure and help us track posture and movement. Plenty of us cope with varying degrees of disconnection from the neck down. It is deceptively easy to confuse judgments about appearance for the actual architecture of our unique form. By locating and identifying the primary landmarks of the body, we learn to see ourselves more clearly and, I hope, appreciatively. We begin body mapping with self-examination and progress toward anatomical touring with fellow body-curious folks.

Once we start to recognize how our bones come together, we will interpret how the body shifts and carries weight in positions that range from seated to standing to supine. Specifically, we will have a gander at a postural and movement paradigm known as the Integrated Model of Function (IMF). This model offers a framework to discern how each of our parts connect to and function in relationship with all the others throughout the body. I like to think of this model as a jumping-off point for any excursion on the mat.

Then we will get on the mat and begin our physical training. To prepare for the rigors of practice, we will learn several functional movement series. The overarching intention of each training series is multilayered: to cultivate attentiveness and sensitivity all the way to the bones, to unravel and rewire movement arrhythmias, and to build foundational strength and mobility to help us explore and grow our asana practice.

We also need to pace ourselves. Any quest ideally includes some downtime to recharge our batteries. Even if we pay lip service to and sincerely understand the power of restorative practices, we most likely will choose to work rather than rest when our time and energy resources are under strain. Take a moment, though, to recall Sir Isaac Newton's third law of motion, which basically states that for every action, there is an equal and opposing reaction. Thus, if we want to improve our chances of bodily comfort and ease of movement, we absolutely need to chill out. At a minimum, our tissues need a respite, especially when challenged by fatigue or injury. Each practice series concludes with meditative rest, and the tutorials in Chapter 7 regarding how and when to apply restorative yoga techniques will help us establish a safe place in which to abide with whatever is alive in us. These rest stops will also give us time to reframe detours and breakdowns as opportunities for self-protection and care.

Etiquette for the Explorer: People Before Poses

An essential truth of practice is that there is no yoga without you. There's an aphorism from the Chandogya Upanishad, a Vedantic text, that sums up a fundamental concept about the nature of being: *Tat tvam asi*, or "Thou art That." Just like there's no pot without clay, the Self and Universe are one and the same. When we grok this idea, we also accept an underlying truth of embodiment: there are no superfluous movements, sensations, or postural adaptations. The body is bioengineered to move, and it will adapt to preserve movement, even in ways that we experience as painful or "bad."

Injuries and chronic conditions layer complexity into any physical training, asana included. Pain and other limitations from, say, a herniated disc, an inflamed tendon, or acid reflux may befuddle our attempts to become more comfortable in body—not to mention in heart, mind, and spirit. We often label our individual adaptations as problematic—for example, "I have a bad knee." As someone who has had parts replaced, repaired, and removed, I know this tendency all too well. The struggle to accept perceived deficits and dysfunctions as they are, rather than how we wish them to be, is real. We walk a tightrope, pushing ourselves further toward the edge of our tolerance, especially when we brand our bodies, efforts, and selves as wrong, bad, or not enough.

A turnaround in self-talk cultivates the willingness to tend and befriend ourselves moment to moment. While reading this book, refrain from using "good," "bad," "right," and "wrong" as descriptors of any aspect of appearance, condition, feeling, or function. Since adjectives are judgments, they are self-limiting and narrowing. Instead, identify the general feeling that gathers your attention. Then notice where you are aware of sensation in the body. For example, you may be upside down in Headstand (Sirsasana) and become attentive to a feeling of anxiety. You may then become aware that you feel emotional tension in your gut or throat. It's not so much a matter of what is alive in you; it's a matter of continuing to delve into the discernible now of aliveness, whatever it is.

Resist the temptation to intellectualize and categorize your feelings and accompanying sensations. Stop yourself from using "feels like" statements. Once you follow the track of "feels like," you've entered contested territory, with its attendant adjectives and adverbs. Feelings and sensations don't feel like anything other than themselves. They're like primary colors: sure, they can be blended to form a multitude of hues and tones, but all those blended colors come from basic types of emotions and bodily sensations. Our feelings are distilled from glad, mad, sad, and scared; our sensations are perceived as pressure, temperature, position, pain, and touch. By training our attention on the taproots of feelings and sensations, we learn to label and track them until they shift. Noticing the shifts helps buy us time, a breath or two at least, before leaping to conclusions. As we practice observing and identifying how and where we feel, we learn to recognize patterns and roadblocks that hold us away from our inner selves.

The shift in language from judgments and analysis to the essence of our feelings and sensations moves us into the wide-open vistas of the present where understanding, empathy, and compassion reveal themselves. As we trek along in search of asana, we encounter innumerable scenic overlooks that offer remarkable views of the relationships within ourselves as well as with family, friends, and so on. It's not unusual to feel some discontent between what we had hoped to see and what is before us.

To bridge the gap between expectation and reality, it helps to observe that every single pose is new to us every single time we practice. The asana has never happened before, whether expressed by different individuals or by the same person multiple times in a sequence. We can also cut across formal definitions about what constitutes asana. Rather than defining its practice as the display of static or "finished" forms, think of asana as a fluid state of abiding in somatosensory inquiry. In this way, we place people before poses, and the asana emerges from us, not over us.

When we step onto the mat, we are taking a leap of faith into the universe within. It's no understatement to proclaim that grand adventures, fraught with risk and rich with reward, await your wonderful self. Let's support your journey with some lessons in mapmaking and navigation.

2

Lay of the Land

BODY LANDMARKS FOR ASANA

It's a dangerous business, Frodo, going out your door.
You step onto the road, and if you don't keep your feet,
there's no knowing where you might be swept off to.
—J. R. R. Tolkien[1]

One of my favorite pastimes is hiking. There have been trails that have literally brought me to my knees, courtesy of a misplaced foot- or handhold. Many a trek has evoked responses to terrain and weather, mindset and health that led me to take a metaphorical knee. Notably, all these adventures require route planning, which means lots of time dedicated to the study of maps. Whether you're heading off into the woods or a city center, maps serve as indispensable travel guides. They encompass a tremendous amount of information, from where and how people live in the context of geography, politics, and economy, to how the earth shapes itself in response to natural forces of the cosmos.

You may be asking yourself what maps and trip planning have to do with asana practice. More than we might consider at first nod! What is asana but a location where we position our awareness to take stock of our relationship with our current internal and external environs? Alignment principles and other ideas about asana practice essentially serve as maps, inviting us to venture into the topographically rich and complex terrain of body, breath, heart, and spirit where each pose is encountered.

In asana, we pick our way along ridgelines and valleys, skeletal and existential, that help shape our experiential territory, seeking stable footholds and solid ground. Once we arrive in the locus we recognize as Mountain Pose, we stay awhile to take in the vistas and feel the air on our skin. We usually encounter new, unexpected Mountain Poses the longer we poke around the vicinity. Asana, thus, trains us to locate our awareness and explore our state of being in situ, a skill that we can take off the mat and into any moment.

Route Planning: Explorations and Excursions

Asana practice, like any sort of journey, is well served by plotting a course, and the study of anatomy is a primary component of route planning on the mat. I must confess, I believe anatomy study supports asana practice as a foundational pillar of yoga education. Evidence-informed, empathy-based, inclusive information about how we are put together and how our parts interact is a precursor to self-care and advocacy on and off the mat.

Anatomy is basically a type of geography that helps us know what we are looking at when we observe ourselves in the mirror. The reality is, the more we learn about a location, the more likely we are to recognize its features and consider how those features are affected by stimuli. That is what we are doing when we map and identify the bony landmarks of the body. We are building an understanding and appreciation of our anatomical geography. The more bodily landmarks we recognize, the better equipped we are to make realistic, safe requests for ourselves in asana.

FOR THE LANGUAGE LOVERS: TECHNICAL TERMS

Just like geography, anatomy has a specialized vocabulary. Consider that we describe mountains as having outcroppings, peaks, and stream channels. Various attributes of our skeletal form have names evocative of the features and terms depicted on topographical maps, such as the *promontory* of the sacrum, *acromion* of the shoulder blade, and external acoustic *meatus* of the ear. We don't have to become fluent in the technical vocabulary of anatomy to formulate a detailed map of our bodies. However, the language of anatomy is full of details we might appreciate as body cartographers. To that end, each bony landmark section has a list of anatomical terms for further study.

Many of us, especially those who lead others in movement, understand so-called normal anatomy and ideal posture as a basis for comparison when watching others sit, stand, walk, or practice Triangle Pose. Even more of us carry subconscious and conscious beliefs that our individual divergences from "normal" and "ideal" might serve as signs that something about our bodies may be wrong or deficient. As a point of fact, a lot of us do have diagnosed and undiagnosed concerns about our anatomy and functioning. However, we can unload some of the worry and gain valuable insight by learning to see, touch, name, and feel our bodily features and sensations. If we do decide to seek care from a licensed health care provider after studying our bony bits and soft-tissue slings, we will be equipped to discuss our concerns based on observation and experience.

FOR THE DARING: DEEPER DIVES

Our body mapping exercise is focused on the major, or primary, bony landmarks of the body. However, different adventures await us off the beaten path. Each bony landmark section includes a detour to connect with local culture. These exploratory excursions offer guided inquiries into additional details of our regional anatomy. Check out these optional forays at your own inclination.

Body mapping is an exercise in self-understanding and empathy. As we proceed, hold this mantra in the forefront of your awareness: everybody is unique, just like everyone else. So, let's hone our surveying skills to follow the lay of the land—its peaks, passages, and pathways—and find the natural landmarks in our own body map.

Surveying Skills: Perspectives, Tools, and Topography

What follows is a body mapping exercise to identify distinctive features of our skeletal anatomy. In later chapters, we will discuss the soft tissues that overlay our bony structures. By focusing our attention on assorted knobs, depressions, gaps, ridges, and crests of the bones, we will distinguish where and how the bones come together as joints, have a clearer sense of proportions, and hopefully feel closer to our bodies than before.

When examining some areas of the body, such as the feet and ankles, we may prefer to scope out the regional anatomy from a comfortable seated position. Otherwise we will examine the body's topography from the perspective of Mountain Pose. For our purposes, Mountain Pose entails standing and facing forward, with the feet placed comfortably. The arms hang naturally by the sides of the body, palms facing forward without force or strain.

You will need to work with a mirror, human or glass, that allows a full-body view and a second mirror, like a handheld one, to reflect the back and sides of the body. Remember, you want to look at yourself—and any consenting partner(s)—from the front, back, left, and right. Why both sides of the body? Because one foot—or arm, leg, or collarbone—may be longer than the other. Furthermore, our bodies frequently display bulkier muscles on one side due to dominant handedness and repetitive motion tasks. By looking closely at the bony landmarks on each side of the body, we may notice patterns in how the forces and residues created by our activities inform our shape. You may want to have your favorite anatomy book, website, or app accessible for reference.

We want to feel bony topography as well as see it, so we will use touch extensively. Since you may not be able to reach some areas, like the midback, you may find that a tennis or springy rubber ball can serve as a free hand. By pinning the ball between your body and a wall, you can move against the wall, and the ball will find the bony bits that stick out and valleys that curve inward.

You may also want to have colored masking tape or adhesive dots on hand. Most folks find it helpful to place a piece of tape or an adhesive dot on each bony landmark. The visual aids highlight how we are put together. You may have difficulty placing the visual markers on the back of your own body. No worries! Mark what and where you can. You will still be able to get the proverbial lay of the land.

Speaking of land navigation, all explorers need a compass to stay oriented. The following list of terms tell us where we are on the body map while standing in Mountain Pose or seated. Think of these terms as compass points indicating the anatomical equivalents of north, south, and otherwise:

Toward or at the front = anterior
Toward or at the back = posterior
Toward or at the top = superior
Toward or at the bottom = inferior
Toward or near the trunk or some major joint = proximal
Away from the trunk or some major joint = distal
Toward the middle or midline = medial
Away from the middle or midline = lateral

Keep in mind that body mapping is not a diagnostic process. It is an educational activity to develop visual, tactile, and sensory fluency with our structure. If any of the touch tactics stimulate physical sensations such as pain, numbness, or tingling, or psychoemotional distress, you might consider following up with a licensed health care provider. Regardless of your findings along the way, undertake the survey with soft eyes, gentle hands, and an open heart.

Mapmaking with Others

Ideally, we want to work in person with several people. Working with more than one person allows us to notice with specificity that everybody is unique. If you are working with others, please state explicitly where, why, and how you would like to touch. Ask—and wait! —for consent. For example, "I would like to find [insert specific landmark] with my fingertips. May I touch [insert specific area]?" We want to cocreate feelings of safety and respect with one another. Sharing information about our intentions and asking for consent goes a long way toward establishing mutuality on (and off) the mat.

Also, there are some areas that we simply do not touch. The groin area and inner thighs are absolutely off limits. Seriously and specifically, we do not touch or stare at the pubic juncture or inner thighs. That's why we do not probe for the lesser trochanter on the inner, upper thigh bone, even though it is an attachment point for the psoas major and iliacus muscles. We also do not look for the front of the hip joints on another person. If you are working with other people, ask *them* to find their own hip joints as instructed in this exercise. Out of respect for the "city of jewels" and breast tissue, avoid touching the belly or front of the rib cage. When seeking the bony landmarks of the rib cage, work from the back body toward the sides rather than standing chest-to-chest with your partner.

Furthermore, please consider that adjectives are expressions of judgment. I rely on observation-based turns of phrase, such as "The left [insert bony landmark name here] feels/looks longer/wider/thicker to me." I try to steer away from comments like "good," "bad," "normal," "abnormal," "*wow*," or even "hm." I learned the socially awkward way to be more cognizant of my language.

Since the feet connect us to the earth, functionally and figuratively, start your observational journey from there. Remember to "pin" the landmarks with a piece of tape or some other marker as you like. Build your anatomy vocabulary by referring to the table of terms at the end of each section.

To help find the body landmarks on yourself or consenting partners, refer to the annotated illustrations at the end of the chapter called Mountain Pose Anatomy Avatars. Each avatar reflects a different view of this pose with circles and ovals indicating where to sight visible and/or palpable landmarks. The avatars show the anterior view (Figure 2.1), posterior view (Figure 2.2), and side view (Figure 2.3) of the body.

Foot and Ankle Topography

Some of us might not be huge fans of the feet from an aesthetic point of view; however, view the feet and ankles through the lens of locomotion. No matter their appearance, these appendages are replete with special formations, detailed in Table 2.1, capable of supporting our weight to and fro.

Landmark 1: Locate the base of the big toe where it meets the long bone of the medial foot. Scan the second, third, and fourth toes. We are just taking in the appearance of the toes.

Landmark 2: Find the base of the little toe where it meets the long bone of the outer or lateral foot. Make note of how much of the toenail is visible. Again, we are simply looking at the toes.

Landmark 3: Feel your way along the little-toe side of the foot until you find a bony knob as you make your way toward the heel. This is the end of the little-toe bone, and it helps us find the beginning of the heel and ankle.

Landmark 4: Next, feel around the bony knob of the inner ankle. This is the bottom end of your shinbone, or tibia. Walk your fingers around the front of the ankle until you feel a channel. To make it easier to find, flex your foot by pulling the forefoot up toward your shin. This channel lies between the shinbone and outer leg bone known as the fibula. Notice how much larger the tibia is compared to the fibula.

Landmark 5: Find the bony knob of the outer ankle. It is formed by the bottom end of the fibula. Work your fingers around the end of the fibula. It feels more like a shield versus a cup for the outer ankle.

TABLE 2.1   Anatomy Terms: Foot and Ankle

BONY LANDMARK DESCRIPTION	TECHNICAL TERM
Base of big toe	First metatarsophalangeal joint formed by proximal phalange and distal end of first metatarsal
Base of little toe	Fifth metatarsophalangeal joint formed by proximal phalange and distal end of fifth metatarsal
Bony knob at ankle-end of little-toe bone	Proximal tuberosity of fifth meta-tarsal
Bony knob on inner ankle	Medial malleolus formed by distal end of tibia
Bony knob on outer ankle	Lateral malleolus formed by distal end of fibula
Shinbone	Tibia
Outer leg bone	Fibula

DEEPER DIVE: FROM TOES TO NECK

There's an adage I know that states, "What happens in the feet happens in the neck." I've encountered this phenomenon more often than I can catalog. So let's take a side trip and explore the kinetic chain from the toes to the neck.

As you examine the feet, notice the distribution of weight. Rock from side to side and toe to heel, then settle into both feet. Feel the pressures within the feet. Pay particular attention to the relationship between the big- and little toe-sides of each foot, and the relationship between the feet themselves.

Look at all the toes. Toe pressure is key to how we push off the earth when we are walking or running. Calluses on the tips of the second toes, along with thickened, tough tissue bumps on the inner edge of the big toes, may indicate overpronation, or the feet rolling inward too much, when walking and running. Check the bottoms of your shoes when you have a chance. You may notice that the wear pattern correlates with the calluses on your toes. Toe pressure is also responsive to pelvis position. If the pelvis is too far forward or behind the ankles and heels, the toes will compensate by gripping or lifting.

Look at the arches on both sides of the feet. Not only do we have an arch across the width of the foot, but we also have two long arches that span the big- and little-toe sides of the feet. Depending on the individual, you may or may not see the smaller arch on the little-toe side of the foot.

We look at the arches because the anatomical reality is that lots of us have flat feet or high arches. Flat or exaggerated arches often mess with the ankles, knees, and hips. These disruptions, in turn, affect the curve of the low back. Lo and behold, the curves of the low back and neck are sympathetic with one another, meaning when one moves, the other naturally tends to follow. In other words, the ability of the arches in the feet to distribute weight and concussive impact while walking or jumping back on the mat translates all the way up to the neck via the superior joints of the legs and curve adjustments in the low back.

Take some time now and expand your attention into the sensations of your body, from the feet all the way into the neck. Experiment with the kinetic chain by shifting your weight in your feet and changing the curve of your low back. Make note of any remarkable details, then return to the main trail. We will explore principles about weight distribution and the like further in this chapter and beyond.

Knee Topography

Move your attention up your legs to your knees. Take a moment and send some gratitude into your knees. The knee is a major confluence between ankle and hip. There's no way you are making it to the mountaintop without learning how to manage those junctions with care. The parts of the knee are identified in Table 2.2.

Landmark 1: Find the big, bony knob at the upper vantage point of the inner, or medial, knee. It is formed by the bottom end of the thigh bone. Without too much pressure, press all around this rounded knob.

Landmark 2: Shift your attention now to the upper, outer knee. Find the smaller bony knob at this end of the thigh bone.

Landmark 3: Switch your attention back to the medial aspect of the knee. From the end of the thigh bone, continue pressing onto the big-toe side of your tibia (also referred to as your shinbone). You will feel a bony thickness that tapers downward. This is the medial aspect of the top of the shinbone. The top of this bone forms two shallow depressions, and the rounded knobs at the end of the thigh bone sit in these corresponding hollows.

Landmark 4: Switch your attention back to the lateral aspect of the knee. From the end of the thigh bone, slide your fingers along the shinbone, slightly toward the front. You will find another bony thickness on the shinbone itself that marks the front edge of the smaller of the two hollows at its top.

A word of caution here: It is easy to confuse the top end of the fibula with the shinbone. It's important, however, to differentiate between the two bones since the fibula is not actually part of the knee joint. Walk your fingers farther around your outer leg from the shinbone. You will feel another bony lump. This is the top end of the fibula. Press around this lump and locate its margins. Then grasp it with your thumb and index fingers. Give it a little wobble from front to back.

Landmark 5: Next, identify the bony shield covering the front of the knee. For comparative purposes, note whether one kneecap looks and feel larger than the other.

Landmark 6: Skim your fingers down the center of the kneecaps onto the front of the shinbones. Just below the kneecaps, feel around until you come upon bony bumps on the front of the tibia, near the top. This is an attachment point for a major knee tendon.

Landmark 7: Last, look at the back of the knee. Typically, we would expect to see a shallow hollow, or "knee pit." With a light touch, skim this area. There is no need to apply pressure, since the arteries, veins, nerves, and lymphatic structures for the lower leg and foot traverse this region. We look at it mainly to familiarize ourselves with the depth of the knee hollow when standing in Mountain Pose.

TABLE 2.2   Anatomy Terms: Knee

BONY LANDMARK DESCRIPTION	TECHNICAL TERM
Bony knob at end of thigh bone	Femoral condyle, medial or lateral, formed by distal end of the femur
Top of shinbone, big-toe side	Medial aspect of the tibial plateau
Top of shinbone, little-toe side	Lateral aspect of the tibial plateau
Bony lump at top of outer leg bone	Proximal head of the fibula
Bony knob at top center of shinbone	Tibial tuberosity
Bony shield or cap covering front of knee	Patella (singular), patellae (plural)
Hollow at back of knee	Popliteal fossa
Thigh bone	Femur
Shinbone	Tibia
Outer leg bone	Fibula

DEEPER DIVE: ACROSS THE GAPS

Knees are complicated because so many forces pass through them. Learning how to cross over the gaps between the thigh bone and shinbone is imperative if you want to stay upright on your feet. Let's scout the crevices and slots of the knee.

Start at the thigh bone's big, bony knob at the top of the inner knee. As before, press gently all around this knob. You will find a gap. This is the space between the medial end of the thigh bone and the top of the shinbone—incidentally, this space is home to a cartilage structure known as the medial meniscus. Continue walking your fingers around to the outer side of the knee, pressing gently around the smaller bony knob at this end of the femur. You will feel a gap here as well, which is where the lateral meniscus resides.

You may notice that the gap on the inside of the knee feels longer and bigger than the one on the outer side. The medial top of the shinbone is larger and its depression deeper, since it meets up with the bigger knob at the end of the thigh bone.

Now, check out your kneecaps. The kneecaps may look or feel like they are being pulled up and out. You may already have instances when your kneecap hitches or gets caught when you straighten your knee. Often, tight, imbalanced, and/or weak quadriceps on the front of the leg, plus ornery iliotibial (IT) bands spanning from outer hip to lower leg (see Chapter 4), require some TLC.

Alternatively, the kneecaps may look or feel like they are drooping down and pressing in. You may know that you are prone to hyperextending your knees. Regardless, make note of patellar positions, since this will help formulate strategies for improving their function in asana.

Hip, Pelvis, and Low Back Topography

Continue your body survey by shifting attention to your pelvis, hips, and lumbar region, with anatomical terms shown in Table 2.3. Be sure to have plenty of adhesive dots or masking tape on hand. Mirrors will come in handy, if available. We will begin by looking at the back body.

Landmark 1: Locate the bony knobs of the outer hip, at approximately the same level as where the thigh bones link into the pelvis. It may be helpful to seek these structures in relationship to the outer seam of your pants legs. In most of us, the knobs sit slightly behind, or posterior to, the seam; however, they may sit right at the seam. Place the tape on these lateral hip structures and proceed with your observations.

Landmark 2: Next, look at the back of your pelvis in the mirror. Place your hands around your back and sides, on the top edge of the large, ear-shaped hip bones. These bony rims form the upper ridgeline of the pelvis.

Landmark 3: Slide your hands along the upper ridgeline of the back pelvis, toward the midline of the body. You will feel the upper part of the angled, wedge-shaped bone—the sacrum—that lives between the hip bones. Work your fingers onto the sacrum to feel its angle. Then walk your fingers away from the midline, until you find your way back to the hip bones. You will feel an angled edge of the hip bones that mirrors the angle of the sacrum. This aspect of the hip bone is akin to the sloping curve of the outer upper ear. Some people have two dimples on either side of the sacrum, which make it easier to find this slope.

Landmark 4: Our last stop on the back of the pelvis is the end of the lumbar spine and uppermost aspect of the sacrum. Place your hands on the crests of the hip bones and again work your thumbs toward the midline of your body. Feel the upper sacrum and then shift your thumbs upward, into the valley of the lumbar spine. This channel is formed by the muscles running alongside the vertebral column. Press inward firmly but judiciously and look for a fingertip-sized bump near the bottom of the low back. This bump marks the end of the bony "finger" that protrudes off the last bone of the lumbar spine.

Landmark 5: Now, turn your attention to the front of the pelvis and belly. Press lightly into or look at your belly button. Your navel sits opposite the disc between the bones of your middle lumbar spine. The body's center of gravity resides approximately two to three finger widths below the belly button.

Landmark 6: Find the "eyes" of your pelvis, which correlate with the bony angle along the front edge of each hip bone. Place your fingers on top of your hip bones at the side waist, then feel down along the top of the front edge of the hip bones, until you come to small, bony knobs. Peekaboo!

Landmark 7: The last marker we place on the front of the pelvis is the location of the hip sockets. Many of us might think of the outer thigh, where the thigh bone meets the pelvis, as the hip joint. Instead, we need to orient ourselves to the true hip joints, which are saucer-like depressions closer to the midline of the body than we might expect. Stand in Mountain Pose and internally rotate your thigh bones a bit. That action should reveal the depressions that indicate the hip sockets.

TABLE 2.3   Anatomy Terms: Hips, Pelvis, and Low Back

BONY LANDMARK DESCRIPTION	TECHNICAL TERM
Bony knob at outer hip, approximately level with pubic bone	Greater trochanter formed by bony eminence, the distal end of the neck of the femur where the shaft of the thigh bone begins
Top, bony rim of back and sides of the large, ear-shaped hip bones	Iliac crest
Thigh bone	Femur
Large, ear-shaped hip bone	Ilium (singular), ilia (plural)
Angled edge on back of hip bones, toward the midline, from top, bony rim down along sacrum	Posterior superior iliac spine (PSIS)
Angled, wedged-shaped bone between hip bones	Sacrum
End of lumbar spine	Lumbar vertebra 5 (L5) of 5 vertebrae (sometimes 6)
Uppermost aspect of sacrum	Sacral vertebra 1 (S1), also called sacral promontory, base of sacrum
Fingertip-like bump that protrudes off back of vertebral bone	End of spinous process (e.g., spinous process of L5)
Bones of middle lumbar spine	Lumbar vertebrae 3 (L3) and 4 (L4)
"Eyes" of the pelvis, or bony bumps on front edge of hip bones	Anterior superior iliac spine (ASIS)
True hip sockets	Anterior aspect of the acetabulum, formed by the ilium, ischium, and pubis bones (aka "pubic bones")

DEEPER DIVE: ELEVATION CHANGES AND BASE CAMPS

As you work your way around the basin of the pelvis, it may become evident that one hip bone is higher than the other. You may also notice that one hip bone appears or feels rolled forward or backward of the other. Rest assured, these shifts in elevation are common, and we can undertake simple adjustments and exercises to work toward balance between the bones in asana. The primary movement series detailed in Chapter 5 offers several options.

One of the first steps we can take to navigate the lifts and shifts of the hip bones is to set up a sheltered base camp. On the mat, the feet form our base camp, and the size or width of this base needs to correlate with the sacrum. The heel-to-arch tightrope so many of us walk in poses like Triangle Pose is inappropriate for many bodies, since it is too narrow to allow healthy, passive joint movements to occur between the sacrum, hip bones, and low back. Instead, we need to figure out the span of our sacrum and adjust our foot placement accordingly. Sacral width is indicated by the space between those angled edges on the back of your hip bones, known as the posterior superior iliac spines.

To get the gist of its width, place a length of masking tape across your sacrum from PSIS to PSIS. Next, experiment with foot placement until you feel a sense of whole-body steadiness. Most of us will feel steadier with our feet placed farther apart rather than standing with the feet close together. Once you find the sweet spot for your feet, place a length of masking tape on the mat from the space between the second and third toes on each foot, to provide a visual reference of the base width. If you are working with other body cartographers, spend some time comparing the width of everyone's sacrum. I guarantee that you will encounter a few surprises and insights.

Spend a lot of time familiarizing yourself with the pelvis. Based on many years of life, practice, and teaching experience, I have long believed the pelvis is the most important region of the body when it comes to postural and movement observation, and thus postural and movement therapeutics. More on that in Chapter 4.

Torso and Shoulder Girdle Topography

Bring your gaze up to your rib cage. There are many reasons why we adjust our posture to protect this region both physically and emotionally. Take your time in this neck of the woods, and refer to the avatars at the end of the chapter. The anatomical terms are listed in Table 2.4.

Landmark 1: Place your hands around the bottom of your rib cage. Trace the ribs to where they connect with the breastbone. Feel how your lower ribs enclose the sides of the belly cavity. The bottom rib you are feeling on your side waist is rib 10.

Landmark 2: From rib 10, feel along the back of your bottom rib cage. Press gently inward to find the two short ribs that do not wrap around the side waist like the ribs higher up. We want to locate these ribs since they provide protective cover to the sensitive kidneys and indicate the end of the thoracic spine. You may find it helpful to place a length of masking tape along the area corresponding to ribs 11 and 12 as well as along the bottom ribs on the side waist.

Landmark 3: Next, direct your attention to the front of your body and rest your fingers lightly on your collarbones. Walk your fingers toward the base of your throat until you come to a pair of bony knobs. These knobby ends indicate where the collarbones meet little notches near the top of the breastbone.

Landmark 4: Follow the collarbones out toward your shoulders with your fingertips. You will find another bony knob at this end of each bone.

Landmark 5: Walk your fingers onto and all around the "shelf" at the top of the shoulder. Shrug your shoulders up and slide them down to feel how the ends of the collarbones attach to this bony outcrop.

Landmark 6: From the bony outcrop at the top of the shoulder, trace your fingers down to your back. Follow the horizontal ridge of bone toward the midline of your body. You are feeling the bony spine near the top of the shoulder blade. If you need a longer reach, try using a ball between your back and the wall to find this structure.

Landmark 7: Track the spine of the shoulder blade until you feel its downward turn. Again, a ball massage can reveal things a bit more clearly. With some pressure, you may feel the upper corner of the shoulder blade—shrugging may help you find this bony angle.

Roll the ball down along the bony edge of the shoulder blade, parallel to the thoracic spine, and around the bottom "wing tip." Keep going along the bony edge and along the side body, up toward the armpit. If you are not using a ball, try swinging your arms to get a sense of the shoulder blade's bony perimeter.

TABLE 2.4 Anatomy Terms: Torso and Shoulder

BONY LANDMARK DESCRIPTION	TECHNICAL TERM
Collarbone	Clavicle
Breastbone	Sternum
Floating ribs	Ribs 11 and 12, of twelve pairs of ribs
End of thoracic spine	Thoracic vertebra 12 (T12), of 12
Bony knob at breastbone end of collarbone	Sternoclavicular joint
Shelf at top of shoulder	Acromion
Bony knob at shoulder end of collarbone	Acromioclavicular joint
Shoulder blade	Scapula (singular), scapulae (plural)
Bony ridge near top of shoulder blade	Scapular spine
Bony edge of shoulder blade, parallel to thoracic spine	Vertebral border of scapula
Bottom wing tip of shoulder blade	Inferior angle of the scapula
Bony edge of shoulder blade, along side of body	Lateral border of the scapula
Fingertip-like bump that protrudes off back of vertebral body	Spinous process (e.g., of T12)
Three places in thoracic spine where there is more movement potential	T4, T8, and T12

DEEPER DIVE: NAVIGATING SPINES

The bony landmarks of the rib cage and shoulders can help us get oriented to the thoracic spine. Since most people have a dominant side, the thoracic region of the body can get overloaded thanks to repetitive motion strain. Plus, there are three places in the thoracic spine where more movement is possible because the thoracic curve itself naturally changes at these spots. So it helps to know where these places are found.

From the spine of either shoulder blade, with your fingers or the ball, track a horizontal line to the spinal column. Gently but firmly press inward and seek the fingertip-like bump sticking off the back of the vertebral column. This bump marks T4, where the thoracic spine begins to stiffen.

Work the ball or your fingers down to the level of the wing tips at the bottom of the shoulder blades. The finger-like protrusion of T8 sits at or just below the wing tips. Here, the thoracic spine starts to become a bit more mobile; it is stiffer from T4 to T8, to protect the back of the heart and its juncture with the lungs.

To find the last spot along this trail, place your hands or the ball on the back of your rib cage to locate bottom ribs 11 and 12. Slide your fingers or the ball gently along these ribs toward the spinal valley at the midline of the body. Press inward to feel the bony fingertip protruding off the last thoracic vertebrae, T12. Familiarity with T12 is valuable because lots of folks experience discomfort here. Many of us habitually initiate bending forward at this spinal segment, which is a tendency that we need to change to save our breath and back.

Head and Neck Topography

The penultimate region of our body mapping invites us to take a closer look at the back of the neck and head, the pinnacle of our terrain. Anatomical terms are defined in Table 2.5.

Landmark 1: Place your hands comfortably at the base of your neck. You will feel a relatively large bony prominence. This spot marks the fingertip-like projections off the bottom bone of the neck and the topmost bone of the thoracic spine.

Landmark 2: Take your fingers to the base of your skull. Feel the rounded, bony "feet" of the skull and space around them. We want to protect this space, especially when lifting the chin, since the blood supply to the brain flows through this zone.

Landmark 3: Sweep your fingers upward and feel the relative flatness of the back of your skull. Above the flat area of bone, you will feel a horizontal ridgeline. As a rule, when in a supine position, you want to rest the weight of your head from this ridge to the flat area of bone without jamming your chin into your throat.

TABLE 2.5   Anatomy Terms: Head and Neck

BONY LANDMARK DESCRIPTION	TECHNICAL TERM
Fingertip-like projection off bottom bone of neck and top bone of thoracic spine	Cervical vertebra 7 (C7) and thoracic vertebra 1 (T1)
Bony "feet" of skull	Base of occipital bone
Back of the skull	Occipital bone
Horizontal ridgeline, back of skull	Occipital ridge

DEEPER DIVE: TRACING ARCS

Neck pain is a common, unwelcome occurrence. To get a sense of how you may be storing tension in your neck and up into your skull, check the curve of your neck with your hands.

Rest both hands comfortably around the back of your neck. Stroke upward to your head and down to the base of your neck. If the arch of the neck feels evenly distributed, then it is likely in its natural, concave curve. Keep your hands in place.

For comparison, bring your chin down toward your throat and feel your neck round into a hump. When you're ready, lift your chin while supporting the weight of your head. Feel the higher arch created in the back of the neck. Bring your chin down to neutral and take several easy breaths. Rest your arms, if needed.

Bring your hands back up to cradle your neck. The curve may feel interrupted. The bottom half of the neck may feel like a small hump, rounding into your hands. As you slide your hands up toward the base of your skull, you may feel a crease in the flesh near the middle of the neck and that the archway at the top of the neck curves higher. A look at your chin in the mirror usually reveals that it is lifted.

There's no need to worry. Get a feel for the shape of your neck, and pay attention to its sensations during the practice series in Chapters 5 and 6. Several of the exercises are intended to yield sensory-soothing effects for the neck in tandem with other gains.

Arm, Wrist, and Hand Topography

We're coming down from the summit of the mountain now. The last region of the body that we will map comprises the arm, wrist, and hand, with definitions given in Table 2.6.

Landmark 1: Start examining your arms at the shoulders. Feel the rounded top of each upper arm bone. You can feel quite a bit of it.

Landmark 2: Work down the arm to the top of the elbow. Grasp the right and left sides of the elbow, where you can feel bony lumps. These rounded lumps mark the bottom ends of the arm bone.

Landmark 3: Feel the bony shield that covers the back of the elbow. It marks the end of the forearm bone that runs down to the little-finger side of the wrist. The bony cover helps protect the so-called funny bone—so-called because it is a nerve, not a bone, and the funny factor is questionable.

Landmark 4: Look at the palm now. Feel around the soft padding on the little-finger side and the thumb side of the palm. Many of the muscles responsible for gripping lie beneath the padding.

Landmark 5: Notice the shallow valley between these pads. Here lies the carpal tunnel, traversed by the median nerve. The median nerve is the major power conduit for the hands.

Landmark 6: Slide your fingers down to the little-finger side of the wrist. Press around. Do you feel a pea-sized bone knot? It marks where the palm side of the hand meets the wrist. It also gets sore if we press on it too hard in poses such as Plank or Downward-Facing Dog.

Landmark 7: Last, turn your attention to the back of your hand and wrist. Press firmly and gently on the little-finger side. You will feel a bony tooth. Press around the bony edge until you feel a slight dip in the back of the wrist. The dip corresponds roughly with the fourth finger line of the hand. You've just felt the wrist end of a forearm bone called the ulna.

Landmark 8: Drag your fingers along the back of the wrist from the dip toward the thumb side of the wrist. You will bump against the relatively large, stumpy end of the other forearm bone called the radius. Think thumbs up for "rad" or "radical," à la Gen X.

TABLE 2.6 Anatomy Terms: Arm, Wrist, and Hand

BONY LANDMARK DESCRIPTION	TECHNICAL TERMS
Shoulder socket for the arm bone	Glenoid fossa
Shoulder joint	Glenohumeral joint
Bony beak of shoulder socket	Coracoid process
Rounded top of arm bone	Humeral head, or head of the humerus
Arm bone (upper arm bone)	Humerus
Bony lumps on sides of elbow	Epicondyles of the humerus
Bony shield covering back of elbow	Olecranon
Soft padding on little-finger side of palm	Hypothenar eminence
Soft padding on thumb side of palm	Thenar eminence
Shallow valley between pads on little-finger and thumb sides of palm	Carpal tunnel
Forearm bone, from elbow to thumb side of wrist	Radius
Forearm bone, from elbow to little-finger side of wrist	Ulna
Pea-sized bony knot on little-finger side of wrist	Pisiform

DEEPER DIVE: POND HOPPING IN THE DEEP WOODS

The arm bone's "socket" is created by shallow, narrow depressions in the side of the shoulder blade, above the armpit and below the bony roof of the shoulder. While the socket itself is on the shallow end of the pond scale, it is located deep in the body. It is covered by thick chest muscles and several layers of shoulder muscles attached in myriad combinations to the arm bone, various parts of the shoulder blade, and the rib cage.

It can be hard to find the socket and a bit uncomfortable as well. Tread with care as you feel around the head of the arm bone. Scout the bone as deeply as you can—into the chest, at and under the front edge. If you can tolerate it, press directly inward, and there will be a bony beak. This beak is another outcropping of the shoulder blade called the coracoid process. Like the bony outcropping that forms the roof of the shoulder, it functions like a handhold to help keep the head of the arm bone in the socket.

Body Map Complete

Now that we have learned to find our way around the lumps, through the hollows, and across the crevices of the body, we can apply our anatomical knowledge to commune with our natural forms. If you were able to work through the body mapping exercise with other folks, you likely noticed that each of your partners presented with gloriously diverse skeletal characteristics. If you worked solo, you may have noticed some things about your own structure that you would like to explore further.

Regardless, recognition of our unique topography allows us to create posture and movement in a manner that nourishes our bodily intuition. The more intuitive we become, the more harmonious we feel on all layers of being. To further support our asana adventures, let's combine our body mapping skills with some more complex navigational techniques.

Meet the Mountain Pose Anatomy Avatars

Use the following illustrations to help land you in the general vicinity of the anatomical landmarks we've discussed—and to test your memory recall. Label each of the circles and ovals with the bony landmarks as you make body maps. Note anything that made it easier or trickier to find structural features. Remember, everybody is wonderfully different, so the avatars are intended as neutral forms in the service of anatomical inclusivity. Take your time traversing the landscape. You can always come back to specific landmarks that elude your initial explorations. When mapping with others, prioritize informed consent, and folks will gladly go along with you to find out more about themselves.

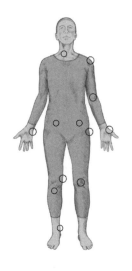 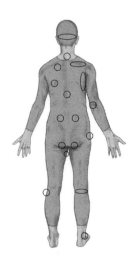 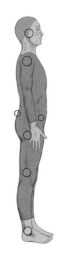

FIGURE 2.1. Mountain Pose Anatomy Avatar, Anterior View

FIGURE 2.2. Mountain Pose Anatomy Avatar, Posterior View

FIGURE 2.3. Mountain Pose Anatomy Avatar, Side View

3

Shaped by Gravity

ANATOMY, MOVEMENT, AND POSTURE

Look deep into nature, and then you will
understand everything better.
—Albert Einstein[1]

We find our way around the body, just like any other location, by following distinctive landmarks that reveal where we are within the specifics of its geography. Akin to signposts, the skeletal landmarks lay out the pathways carved by each person's postural and movement patterns. Some factors that influence our positional attitude and maneuverability are environmental and universal, like gravity. Others are unique and definitively local, shown in each body's shape and physical attitude.

When we recognize the intersection of forces, natural and contrived, in our own structure's static and active states, we become more astute in perceiving the divergences between our needs and circumstances. The temptation to make a beeline for the tourist traps of "alignment" and "normal" might be strong. Their allure is certainly juiced up with all manner of inducements, including the belief that more work, range of motion, and rules compliance are necessities to achieve correct asana.

On the mat, though, we cultivate harmony and balance when we make the asana journey ours and ours alone. In other words, we thrive when we calibrate the relationship between effort and ease. A brief review of some facts pertaining to the physics of embodiment may offer inspiration for revamping the effort-ease interplay.

Forces of Nature: Gravity and Motion

Posture is a direct expression of our relationship with the big G—gravity. Gravity is always pulling downward, and the power of its pull is linked to mass. The denser the mass, the stronger the pull toward the center of the earth. The adage "The bigger they are, the harder they fall" is an apt summation of the relationship between gravity and mass. In the body, this means that its anatomically heavier regions, like the pelvis, are more attractive to gravity. Hence the need in Plank Pose (Chaturanga) for enthusiastic abdominal engagement to hold the pelvis—and head—up against gravity rather than letting them sag downward.

Keep in mind that gravity itself doesn't care if we are standing on our feet, head, or hands, or any combination thereof. All it knows is that there's a body of mass (the human body) close enough to another body of mass (the planet) to make attraction inevitable. That said, our bodies most certainly know which parts are coping with gravity and in what direction. We have built-in somatosensory and control networks that interpret gravity's influence and lead to all kinds of responses by the body's various systems.

The body has its own type of GPS ("gravity positioning system"), known as proprioceptive senses, relating to the different forces within and around it. Assorted monitoring teams are constantly scanning for changes in overall body position, shape, movement, and muscle forces. Proprioceptive senses also process information about the position of the limbs—in relation to one another and the trunk—as well as feelings of strain, heaviness, and the like. For example, receptor bodies in the hamstring tendons keep tabs on load tolerance in Standing Forward Bend and signal whether muscle groups need to behave differently to redistribute work.

Other proprioceptive lookouts sense torque within joints, such as during a biceps curl. Receptors from the wrist to the elbow gauge twisting forces throughout the forearm and rally soft-tissue partners to hold the weight steady through the movement arc. Changes in the positional relationship between the head, heart, and pelvis result in a whole slew of responses. For example, when the head is below the heart, all manner of systems are talking back and forth, from spinal reflexes and muscle activation patterning to blood pressure calibration.

Working in groups, extensive networks of specialized receptors in the skin, joints, and connective tissues, as well as within the respiratory, circulatory, and gastrointestinal systems, automatically send information from the body to a map stored in the brain. This centralized body map is called the homunculus, or "little person." The little person then makes the calls for the "big person," meaning the body, to get with the gravity program in session.

As gravity continuously pulls us downward, other forces are also at play. In terms of asana practice, the forces that garner significant attention are those exerted by muscles. Muscular forces are known as contact forces because two surfaces are involved in the physical interaction. Sometimes we push against surfaces to drive the body and an object away from each other. When we perform a push-up, for instance, we exert a driving force against the earth. Sometimes we pull to drag the body and an object toward each other. When we perform a bent-over rowing motion, we are pulling the arms close to the body.

Different energies further affect changes in speed and shape. Friction is a type of resistance between two surfaces. It serves to decelerate, or slow things down. For example, the textured surface of a yoga mat creates grip, or friction, to reduce slippage. Pressure is the ratio of any type of force to the area over which it is acting vis-à-vis resistance. Thus, pressure may increase to overcome resistance, or it may decrease to preserve flow or motion. On the mat, pressure concerns us when we are positioning joints and practicing pranayama. We simply want to be aware that changes in pressure within our joints and body cavities often indicate where we have too much or too little resistance.

The primary takeaway here is that our bodies develop in response to gravity as well as the forces within and around them. From bone density to spinal curves and reflexes, we grow in ways that allow us to move with and against the constant downward tugging. When observing posture, we are essentially seeing each person's organizational adaptations to living earthbound. Thus, it behooves us to establish some baselines for comparison. Specifically, we want to understand commonly agreed-on benchmarks for so-called normal posture in Mountain Pose. Then we can dissect how local influences, like the type of work performed by an individual, play out in each person's body.

DEEPER DIVE: GRAVITY-INSPIRED GROWTH

The body's growth and movement development are yoked to gravity. Human babies are born with some three hundred bones and cartilaginous structures. Of course, one of the reasons babies come into the world with squishier skeletons is to make the birth process easier. Over time, though, it's the compressive and resistive forces of gravity that will encourage those bones and cartilages to fuse and ossify into the 206 many of us are most familiar with.

Several baby-toddler-child developmental milestones illustrate the union between gravity and our skeletal structure. To start, we join the world of gravity without all of our spinal curves. We are born with a primary, or C-curve, which means kyphosis of the thoracic and sacral regions. We develop the secondary, or S-curves, of the vertebral column as we get used to being landlubbers. The concave, or lordotic, curve of the neck develops as babies gain the strength to lift and turn their heads at around three to six months of age. The lordotic curve of the low back emerges in older babies as they begin to crawl. The lumbar curve continues to develop as young ones gain the ability to walk and run about, from age twelve months onward. The S-curves distribute the force of gravity evenly throughout the body, so retire the old dictum to "stand up straight" and embrace your contours.

Additional developmental milestones improve the efficiency and power of walking, running, and jumping. From ages two to twelve years or so, several cartilage structures turn to bone, or undergo ossification. Specifically, sesamoid bones harden from cartilaginous "sesame seeds" in the flexor tendons of the knees and big toes. The cartilage seeds grow into kneecaps and pairs of "corn kernels" on the underside of the big toes to exert more power with greater efficiency as little feet and legs get to roaming. Kids also grow a couple of sesamoid bones in the hands as they develop grip and dexterity. Of course, our bones grow and harden with age as well. Without being remotely inappropriate, spend some time with family and friends' wee ones to observe these developmental milestones. We all grow at our own rate, so remember our mantra.

Get on the Grid: Vertical and Horizontal Body Lines

We've already familiarized ourselves with the anatomical landmarks that we will use to read the terrain of posture and, later, movement. Now we will lay in some imaginary grid lines on our body map, from the perspective of Mountain Pose, to help us identify divergence from latitudinal and longitudinal average. These lines of reference are vertical and horizontal axes envisioned through the prominent bony landmarks, which can be used to orient ourselves in the frontal, sagittal, and transverse planes.

A plumb line is used as a vertical reference to determine if a structure—the body as a whole and/or specific joints—is aligned in relationship to the perceived center of gravity. Center of gravity (CoG) refers to the area of the body where its mass appears concentrated. In the body, this conceptual center sits above the bladder, at the approximate level of the second sacral segment. On the outer body, the CoG corresponds to three finger widths below the navel in the average female-bodied person, and two finger widths for the average male-bodied person. That said, male-bodied people typically have more mass in their chests and shoulders, so the CoG is functionally much higher in the center of the chest. Keep in mind, CoG is a referential idea, so there's no need to get supertechnical about pinning its location. A sense of where mass seems or feels concentrated is sufficient when it comes to postural interpretation.

A horizontal line is used as a reference to determine if a structure or feature is distributed evenly from right to left, left to right, in relationship to a surface. The line where a wall and floor meet, for instance, is a horizontal line, the same as where the sky and sea meet at the beach. For our purposes, the horizontal grid lines of postural observation run parallel to the floor and perpendicular to the plumb lines.

Since we are adding more detail to our body maps, you may want to have lightweight string and adhesive tape or dots on hand. As before, we will use these visual aids to correlate our features with these orientational lines. Each section also concludes with a table of terms to summarize frequently encountered characteristics.

If you are relying on the illustrations that follow, you will want to consider them as representative rather than technical, as a guidepost for the real deal on the mat. You may also want to do image searches online for comparative purposes. And rest easy! You will regularly get caught in the space of uncertainty when studying the human form; embrace it, my friends, for we grow and learn only in that space.

OBSERVER HACK: HOMEMADE VISUAL AIDS

To help visualize whether a vertical line is straight, fashion a plumb bob. A plumb bob is basically a weighted line used to clarify the levelness of an upright surface. All you need are a couple of common household materials: a 6-foot (2-meter) length of string, a pencil, and three to five heavy washers or a fishing weight.

Tie the washers or fishing weight on one end of the string. Tie the other end of the string securely to the middle of the pencil. Voilà! You now have a basic plumb bob. The pencil serves as the handle and spool. You adjust the length of the plumb bob by wrapping more of the string neatly around the center of the pencil. You can also adjust the position of the line itself along the length of the pencil, to make it easier to hold steady depending on the vertical alignment you would like to assess.

Either looking in a mirror or observing a partner, we hold the ends of the pencil so that the weighted string hangs down from whatever point of reference is the focus. We then look at the weight to see if it swings directly down the center of our plumb line or if it swings to one side or another. For example, by placing the eraser end of the pencil at the center of the bridge of the nose, we can see the overall verticality of the body. To see the verticality of the knees and legs, we hold the pencil evenly in front of the top level of the pubic bones, so the bob displays the vertical line down to the floor.

Keep in mind that we are not seeking mathematical precision. The purpose of a plumb bob, as well as the imaginary grid lines themselves, is to orient ourselves more easily within breathing distance of somatosensory awareness and understanding.

The Body's Primary Grid

When labeling posture and movement, we work within conceptual planes that divide the body along vertical, horizontal, and diagonal slices. Keep in mind, these lines can be innumerable, partitioning the body into a veritable slide show of segments. These planes of motion help us orient ourselves—from head to toe and down to small, individual joints—in space. Refer to Table 3.1 to review the nuts and bolts of deciphering body and movement orientation.

TABLE 3.1 Planes of Motion with Associated Movements and Grid Lines

PLANE OF MOTION	ASSOCIATED MOVEMENTS	GRID LINE
Median (midsagittal)	Flexion, extension	Median (midsagittal, midline, gravitational)
Transverse (horizontal, transaxial, axial)	Rotation	Horizontal (axial)
Frontal (coronal)	Lateral flexion/side-bending, abduction, adduction	Coronal (midaxillary, frontal, gravitational)
Oblique (diagonal)	Combined/compound movements	Oblique (diagonal)

We first sight the reference lines in Mountain Pose. With practice, we then can make inferences about our relationship with gravity in any posture or movement. From weight distribution to the direction of gaze and muscle bulk, we can also make some guesses about our structural harmony, for example, noting differences between the right and left, front and back, and side views. Refer to the Planes of Motion Avatars to visualize your own grid lines.

Also, to help us think in movement terms, the Planes of Motion Avatars are paired with an example of the movements that occur in the plane. Each figure shows a different reference line to orient the body in space. Let's find our latitudes and longitudes!

Primary Grid Line 1: Look at your and/or a consenting partner's full body from the front and back. Imagine a vertical line that divides the body evenly into right and left sides. It bisects the interior spaces of the body too and reveals the balancing act between the head, chest, belly, and pelvic cavities. Known as the primary gravitational line, this is the main plumb line of the body as a whole. It demarcates the midsagittal plane of motion, which relates to flexion and extension movements. A plumb bob comes in handy to clearly view the midline and the body's relationship with it. Refer to Figures 3.1 and 3.2.

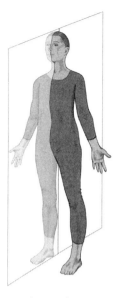

FIGURE 3.1. Planes of Motion Avatar,
Midsagittal Plane

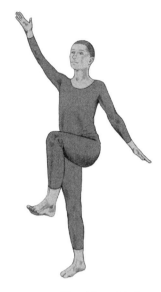

FIGURE 3.2. Marching with Arm
Movements

Primary Grid Line 2: Continue to view the body from the front. Sight a horizontal line at the level of the belly button and carry that line through the back body. Situated as the transverse plane, this line divides the body into top and bottom halves. It serves as a reference for rotational movement, such as a turned rib cage or pelvic girdle. Refer to Figures 3.3 and 3.4.

Primary Grid Line 3: Turn to the side, if you are working solo with a mirror, or walk around to view the side of your partner's body. Visualize another vertical line through the center of the body, which divides it into front and back halves. This gravitational plumb line marks the frontal or coronal plane of motion. It relates to side-bending, as well as moving the limbs toward (adduction) or away from (abduction) the midline of the body. The frontal line also orients elevation and depression of the shoulder blades and jaw. Refer to Figures 3.5 and 3.6.

Primary Grid Line 4: Look at the front body again, and overlay a pair of intersecting diagonal lines. Imagine one line from the center of the right shoulder to the center of the left hip, and a second line

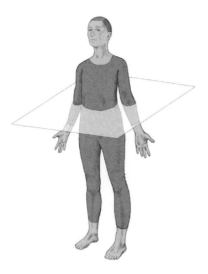

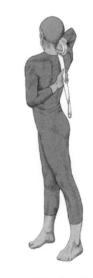

FIGURE 3.3. Planes of Motion Avatar, Transverse Plane

FIGURE 3.4. Standing Twist with Cow Face Arms

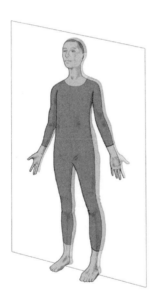

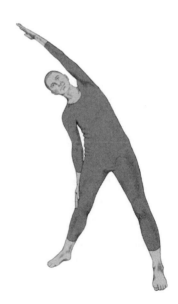

FIGURE 3.5. Planes of Motion Avatar, Frontal Plane

FIGURE 3.6. Wide-Leg Standing Side Bend

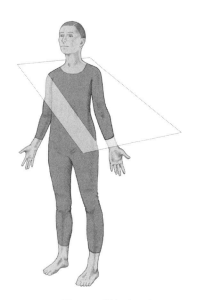

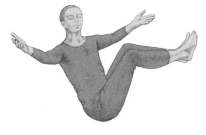

FIGURE 3.7. Planes of Motion Avatar, Oblique Plane

FIGURE 3.8. Revolved Boat Pose

from the left shoulder to the right hip. These lines form an X that intuits the major oblique planes of motion, where compound movements are interpreted. A sample compound movement would be rotation and extension, like turning the trunk and neck to look up and back over the shoulder. Refer to Figures 3.7 and 3.8.

With an overall idea of postural disposition, we now turn our attention to the alignment of the major bodily segments. To stay on the map, we need to see where we are starting at a street-level view. Examination of our interconnected regions in the context of smaller, "neighborhood" grids enables us to pinpoint local digressions from the vertical plumb and horizontal level. By recognizing the individual's characteristics, we learn to correlate and accommodate asana with the shapes expressed from each person's body.

Now is a good time to remind ourselves that symmetry is an illusion, and everyone is different, just like everybody else. To that end, each of the following sections includes a table that lists common variations in our skeletal stacks and postural expressions. For each anatomical region, refer to the Grid Line Avatars (Figures 3.9, 3.10, and 3.11) at the end of the chapter to sight the regional lines from the front, back, and side views of Mountain Pose.

The Foot and Ankle Grid

The next set of grid lines applies to the feet from the ankles to the toes, with anatomical differences defined in Table 3.2. We will assess the symmetry of the toes, feet, and ankles from left to right, and from both the front and back of the body.

Grid Line 1: From the back body, visualize a horizontal line between the inner anklebones (medial malleoli). Within the typical range, these bony knobs appear level with one another.

Grid Line 2: From the back of the body, visualize a second horizontal line between the outer anklebones (lateral malleoli). Sight this line approximately a finger width lower than the first. The outer anklebones appear level with each other on this lower line.

Grid Line 3: Next, also from the back of the body, drop a plumb line from a point of reference above the ankles to the floor. Note the distance between the inner anklebones from this vertical line. Sometimes the inner ankles appear to list toward the midline or drop outward. Similar to knock-knees and bowlegs, you may notice knock or bow ankles.

Grid Line 4: Continue to examine the back of the feet and ankles. Look at the heels and Achilles tendons. Lay another plumb line along the tendons. Ideally, weight is distributed evenly through the heel cup, and the Achilles tendons are vertical. Once again, these tendons, like ankles or knees, may look bent toward the midline (knock foot) or curved outward (bow foot).

Grid Line 5: Change your vantage point and walk around to the front body, either literally or figuratively. Visualize a vertical line between the feet. Look at the position of the toes and make note of the directional orientation—pointing forward or turning inward or outward, from the midline.

TABLE 3.2 Anatomical Terms: Common Variations of the Ankles, Feet, and Toes

COMMON VARIATION DESCRIPTION	TECHNICAL TERM
Ankles that bend inward toward the midline (knock ankles)	Pes valgum
Ankles that bend outward from the midline (bow ankles)	Pes varus
Achilles tendons that bend inward toward the midline (knock feet)	Calcaneovalgum
Achilles tendons that bend outward from the midline (bow feet)	Calcaneovarus
Little to no discernible arch (flat foot)	Pes planus
Elevated, cave-like arch (high arch)	Pes cavus
Second, third, or fourth toe(s) that flexes sharply at the second joint of the toe itself, causing the toe to pull upward and curl under (hammertoe)	Contracted toe
Big toe that bends away from the midline toward the smaller toes, with a bony bump formed where the joint sticks out (bunion)	Hallux valgus

DEEPER DIVE: FLATS AND CAVES

As you observe the position of the toes, heels, and ankles, be sure to take a leisurely perusal along the arches of the feet. If there is little to no discernible longitudinal arch along the big-toe side, this is a flat foot. The effects of the flattened arch will often carry into knock ankles and feet, so consider the feet in relationship to the ankles.

On the other hand, you may notice elevated, cave-like arches, which are called high arches. Hammer- or claw toes may partner with those elevated arches, so make note of any toes that are pulling upward and curling under. Such toes—usually the second toe—resemble the end of a hammer.

Get to know what folks' feet, toes, and ankles look like. It is essential to train the feet as they are integral to healthy movement. Later, we will practice exercises for the feet as well as consider positioning adjustments from foot to hip to feel balanced and stable when practicing standing asana.

The Knee Grid

Knees are a frequent site of vigilance. From Warrior II and Hero Pose (Virasana) to going down a set of stairs, many of us experience aches and pains in the knees. Some of us live with knees so creaky that our days of sneaking around like teenagers breaking curfew are long gone. Knee condition—repaired, rehabbed, chronic, or otherwise—is a powerful variable that affects the movement and positioning choices we make.

Grid Line 1: Drop a plumb line between the knees. Make sure you look at the plumb line from the front and back. To add further complexity to an already challenging functional zone, it is quite common to see folks with knees that diverge toward or away from each other, as noted in Table 3.3. It may be easier to tell from the posterior view that one knee diverges more or less from the plumb line than the other. It's useful to note the vertical stacks of the knees, since you get an immediate idea of a person's single-leg balance. After all, it's easier to balance on a carrot than a banana!

Grid Line 2: From the back, you also want to visualize a horizon line from knee to knee. One knee may look higher than the other. It could be that you or your partner is bending one knee for some reason. We note the knees' horizontal relationship because we may need to work a little differently in asana—for example, by using mat scraps as lifts or placing the feet asymmetrically—to facilitate harmony between the knees.

Grid Line 3: From each side of the body, envision a plumb line to mark the border between the front and back. The knees may appear well centered, divided evenly front to back, with a shallow hollow at the back. Such a knee is called "straight." Some knees may appear noticeably bent, with a deeper back pocket. Alternatively, the knees may appear to be bulging backward, which is called "hyperextended." Leave no stone unturned!

TABLE 3.3 Anatomical Terms: Common Variations of the Knees

COMMON VARIATION DESCRIPTION	TECHNICAL TERM
One or both knees appear bent toward the midline (knock-knees)	Genu valgum
One or both knees appear bent away from the midline (bowlegs)	Genu varum

DEEPER DIVE: STEEP CLIMBS

Female-bodied persons are more likely to be members of the knock-knee club than male-bodied people due to obstetrics-friendly pelvises. Thanks to the biological predisposition toward pregnancy and vaginal childbirth, female knees are more likely to have a steeper climb to and from the hip along a line known as the Q angle. Basically, a uterus-holding body is often wider at the hip and narrower at the knee.

Q angle refers to a diagonal line measured between the tendinous insertion of the quadriceps (primarily the rectus femoris) at the hip and the patellar tendon attachment at the tibial tuberosity, which is compared to the vector measured between the center of the kneecap and the tibial tuberosity. Please remember that this is generalization. There are female-bodied individuals who are bowlegged and male-bodied folks that are knock-kneed. Also, taller people with longer thigh bones tend to have steeper Q angles. We simply want to know the overarching tendencies so as not to overlook details that will impact how we adjust resistance and position to improve joint stability.

The Pelvic Grid

We now apply grid lines to the pelvis, which is like a soup bowl that tips slightly forward without sloshing, much less spilling, its contents. Note that the mild anterior tilt mirrors the convex (kyphotic) curvature of the sacrum and the transition into the concave (lordotic) curve of the low back at S1/L5. So long as there is no pinching sensation at the base of the lumbar spine or discomfort anywhere around the low back and hip region, the tilt is at its natural angle.

Otherwise, our attention is directed toward the level lines between the prominent bony landmarks of the pelvis, like the iliac crest and greater trochanters. We are looking for divergences from horizontal balance as well as any rotation in the pelvic position, defined in Table 3.4.

Grid Line 1: Visualize a vertical line through the pubic symphysis (the middle of the pubic bone). There's no reason to stare if you are looking at another person's body. Look for the midline and move on. We can figure out how an individual's pelvis is positioned via other, less intrusive visual reference points.

Grid Line 2: Run a level line through the greater trochanters. Survey the lines where the thighs join the pelvis. Make a note if one side appears higher than the other.

Grid Line 3: Envision a line across the ASIS. You may want to place dots on these structures to get a clearer sense of their location. Again, note if one side appears higher than the other.

Grid Line 4: Move around to the back body and imagine a level line along the bottom of the buttocks.

Grid Line 5: Next, survey the horizon line across the top of the pelvis, along the iliac crest. One hip bone may appear pulled higher than the other, indicating a hitch in the ilium. One side of the bum may be more visible than the other, say, with more of the right buttock seen from the midline of the body to the outer hip than the left.

Grid Line 6: Last, move your gaze to the sides of body, placing a vertical plumb line from the center of the side chest just behind the center of the greater trochanter. This line divides the pelvis in the frontal plane. As you compare the right and left sides of the body, pay particular attention to the ASIS. For instance, you may notice as you look at the right side that you see the surface contour of the left ASIS. Then, when you look at the left side of the body, you don't see any of the right ASIS. A cross-check reveals that the pelvis is turned toward the right.

TABLE 3.4 Anatomical Terms: Common Variations of Pelvises

COMMON VARIATION DESCRIPTION	TECHNICAL TERM
One hip bone is higher than the other	Upslip of the ilium
One greater trochanter is higher than the other	Leg length inequality
One side of the pelvis appears pulled forward or backward	Pelvic rotation or torsion

DEEPER DIVE: NATURAL TILTS

The pelvis tilts forward or backward along the transverse axis of the hips, its ends marked by the greater trochanters. We feel the directional movements of posterior and anterior tilt when we practice Cat-Cow Pose (Marjaryasana-Bitilasana) or Pelvic Rocking. When we return to neutral pelvic position, note that the sacrum is not positioned vertically or directly up and down.

The sacrum itself is not a vertical bone. It curves forward at its top, which is conversely called the base. The ilia hug the contoured edges of the sacrum, forming the sacroiliac joint where the bones are snugged together with many layers of strong connective tissue. The articulating surfaces, albeit irregular, are enrobed in thin cartilage to allow just enough slide and glide to move a couple of degrees north, south, east, west, north- to southeast, and north- to southwest.

To find your own neutral pelvis, stand at an outer corner of a wall or in a doorway. Adjust your heels, knees, and hips directly under your body. Center your back body along the edge of the corner or doorjamb.

Comfortably rest the back of your head against the edge while gently lifting the base of the skull to adjust your chin and gaze toward level—no force or strain; we're simply moving in the direction of level. Most of us need a thin block or rolled towel at the occipital ridge to achieve a level chin and gaze. Use these props to experiment with your head position.

Rest your spine against the corner's edge from the top to bottom of the shoulder blades. Pull the front bottom ribs comfortably downward to relax any forward rib thrust. You may feel the back of the rib cage lift up and off the low back, offering more breathing room for the kidney zone.

Last, align the center of your sacrum from the beginning of its convex curve near the base down to the start of the tailbone, where it begins to turn under. For most of us, the start of the tailbone begins near the top of the "butt crack." The inner cavities of the body should feel balanced in relationship to one another, like rounded stones stacked into a cairn that marks the path to groundedness.

The Upper Body Grid

As we move upward into the trunk, along the main channel of the vertebral column, we are looking for each person's natural S-curves. We note any sideways deviation of the spine from the midline. We also note any rotation in the rib cage, a head tilt or turn, or unevenness between the shoulders. Table 3.5 defines these variations.

Grid Line 1: Extend a plumb line through the center of the vertebrae, all the way from the crown of the head. Imagine this line running vertically through both the front and back body. When looking at the back body, note the distance of the shoulder blades from the spine and whether the head appears tilted to the side.

Grid Line 2: On the back body, imagine a horizon line—or apply tape lines, if working with a partner—across rib 10 on both sides. Note whether one side of the rib cage appears higher than the other. In such instances, you may infer that your posture partner is side-bent through the lumbar and/or thoracic spinal regions.

Grid Line 3: Sight a level line across the inferior angles of the scapulae, which is also the approximate location of both ribs 7. If one inferior angle is higher than the other, this may indicate an imbalance in the soft tissue around the shoulder blades themselves or a side-bend in the lumbar or thoracic regions. Compare this line with the horizon line across the ribs 10. A cross-reference helps us differentiate regional imbalances in the relationship between the shoulder blades, rib cage, and vertebral column.

Grid Line 4: Take a look at the back of the head again and lay in a level line along the occipital ridge. Ideally, the head appears balanced. If one side of the neck seems shorter and tighter than the other, it might result from a disruption of the vertebral curves. Alternatively, it may be that one shoulder's musculature is tighter and hiking upward toward the ear without observable distortion from the midline.

Grid Line 5: Walk or turn around to the front body. Visualize sagittal plumb lines through the front-center of the shoulder, at the acromioclavicular joints, past the hips. Look at the arms hanging alongside the body with the palms facing forward—which means that the forearms are supinated—and notice their drape.

Each of us displays a carrying angle at the elbow that gives us the space between the hands and side body necessary to swing our arms when walking without hitting our outside hip as well as to carry things with straight arms. The greater the distance between the hands and side body, the steeper the individual's carrying angle. Again, one arm may be closer to the body due to shoulder tension or a divergence in the spinal curves.

Grid Line 6: Most of us are familiar with the commonly projected gravitational line that runs from head to foot via the earlobe, bodies of C1-C5, acromion process of the shoulder, middle of the trunk, just behind the greater trochanter, and slightly anterior to the center of the outer knee and ankle. What we are looking for is any deviation forward or behind this plumb line. A visual perusal of the coronal plane provides valuable information regarding the individual's spinal curves, such as flattened or exaggerated lordosis and kyphosis, and any rotational discrepancies in the pelvis, rib cage, and head.

DEEPER DIVE: FREE THE SPINAL FLOW

It is fairly common to notice flattened vertebral curves. So many of us have been instructed to "open the chest" that we live in a perpetual state of retracted shoulder blades, flattened upper and midback, flared front ribs, and forward head position. Combine that with our bias toward flat bellies, achieved by sucking the belly button inward and upward, and we frequently see a posteriorly tilted or tucked pelvis as well.

When considering postural attitude from the side body, we think in terms of flow: follow the fluidity of the spinal curves, especially where transitional segments lie at L5/S1, T12/L1, C7/T1, and the base of the skull. If you sense any breaks or sharpness where the curves flow into one another, you will want to work to smooth out the transitions. Fortunately, much of the mat training in Chapter 5 is well suited to freeing the spinal flow.

Also, pay exquisite attention to how much of the shoulder you see in relationship to the frontal plumb line. When surveying the pelvis from the side body, we gauged how much of the flank was apparent so we could guesstimate about pelvic torsion. This time, apply the same principles to the shoulder girdle.

You will see more of the back of the right shoulder and rib cage if the person is torqued leftward, and more of these structures on the left side if the shoulder girdle is winding around to the right. A turned rib cage may accompany scoliosis. Regardless, we will work to derotate the shoulder girdle and rib cage in service of the vertebral column.

TABLE 3.5   Anatomical Terms: Common Variations of the Trunk, Neck, and Upper Extremity

COMMON VARIATION DESCRIPTION	TECHNICAL TERM
A sideways and rotational deviation of the natural spinal curves	Scoliosis
A confused neck that appears bent forward in the middle with the chin lifted	Forward head
A rounded convex or backward curve of the spine, e.g., in the upper back/thoracic spine (sometimes called a hunched back)	Hyperkyphosis
A deepened concave or forward curve of the spine, e.g., in the low back/lumbar spine (swayback)	Hyperlordosis
A flattened or reduced concave or forward curve of the spine, e.g., in the neck/cervical spine (military neck)	Hypolordosis

The neck is often an area of complaint for people, especially those who spend long periods driving desks and vehicles. From the side body, we can see if the cervical lordosis is reduced, often called "military neck" or "confused." A confused neck results in a forward head position, which arises from lower cervical vertebrae stuck in flexion and upper vertebrae in extension. There will be a pronounced line of compression in the midneck at C3/C4.

You will typically see a distinct hump at the base of the neck, as well as reduced shoulder flexion and neck rotation. When raising the arms overhead, a person with a forward head will hit a sticky zone at the base of the neck and upper thoracic spine. The imbalance in the neck will also inhibit turning the head. To achieve full range of motion, the person will need to lift their chin as they turn their head, to "leap over" the compression block in the mid-neck.

Cartography Complete: You Are Here!

Thanks to our familiarity with the bony landmarks, we have now laid in the reference lines to create a detailed map of bodily attitude and major joint positions in Mountain Pose. We see where the switchbacks, gullies, and slopes are formed by the body's shape and interactions with gravity. Examining ourselves in the context of vertical and horizontal lines allows us to develop a lens through which to view the functional overlays of our activities of daily living. It also allows us to become cognizant of emotional energies expressed within the dynamic constructs of postural alignment.

Based on this customized map, we can make decisions about the trails we will navigate toward *sthira sukham asanam* (balancing ease with effort). In the near term, we will use the information to engage with the neuromuscular training exercises detailed in Chapter 5. These conditioning series are intended to create foundational harmony for asana practice. Specifically, the exercises are designed to improve functional robustness and reduce strain and risk, whether you have an injury, stamina concerns, or would like to resolve nagging issues or tics in your current practice. Before we get to the mat work, though, we need to explore how we carry loads and transfer energy or force through the body. This necessitates a thorough immersion in the home base of the body—the pelvis.

Meet the Grid Line Avatars

We return to the perspective of Mountain Pose to visualize the vertical and horizontal reference lines and see how the body is stacked and balanced. First, view the body head to toe from the front, back, and side. Then focus your attention on each body region, starting from the foot and ankle and slowly climbing to the head, neck, and shoulders. Use the following illustrations to compare the right and left, front and back, upper and lower parts of the body in relation to limbs, as well as closely connected and farther-flung friends and neighbors. Label the grid lines according to the major bony landmarks they cross. Each horizontal and vertical line corresponds to the regional and whole-body alignment stacks described in this chapter.

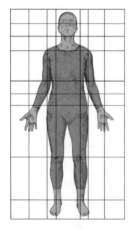 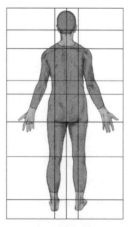 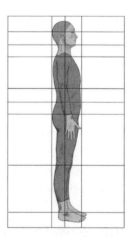

FIGURE 3.9. Grid Line Avatar, Anterior View

FIGURE 3.10. Grid Line Avatar, Posterior View

FIGURE 3.11. Grid Line Avatar, Side View

4

Body in Motion

THE PELVIS POINTS NORTH

We don't reach the mountaintop from the mountaintop.
We start at the bottom and climb up. Blood is involved.
—Cheryl Strayed[1]

Those of us who persist on the mat, especially the longer we grow in practice, are bolstered regularly by a feedback loop of immediate and cumulative effects. After some thirty years of asana practice, I still marvel daily at discoveries unearthed in my somatosensory excursions. Furthermore, the habits of self-reflection engendered by meditative training offer infinite opportunities to recognize evolutions in previously held patterns and beliefs—neuromuscular and otherwise. Taking stock through the lens of consistent, attentive practice usually leads to a sense of relief and healing with contentment, or *samtosha*.

Many of us who teach are drawn to the front of the class as an act of reverence for the revelatory gifts unwrapped along the Eightfold

65

Path of Yoga. Our resonance with the ethical precepts, organizing philosophies, and daily rituals of yogic living is matched in equal measure by the empathy and compassion we nurture with our fellow asana adventurers, also known as the community, or *sangha*. If you've ever attended a yoga class, you may have sensed the threads of mutual courtesy and warm regard woven among the group.

As a teacher-practitioner, I learn something different from every single student I talk with or observe in class. The prevalence of uniqueness has induced me to move further away from prescribed depictions of asana in search of organic postural and movement rhythms. Sometimes there's the merest hint of a passage into Triangle Pose; at other times, the pathways are well traveled. My preferred approach to route-planning and adventure-seeking on the mat is to apply the Goldilocks principle: in the range of each asana, determine the margins between too hard, too soft, and the middle. Then rely on time, patience, and repetition in such a way that everyone can find their experience of "just right."

Meet in the Middle: The Integrated Model of Function

The assessment criteria that comprise my Goldilocks meter arise from an observational paradigm that I have relied on for many years: the Integrated Model of Function. The IMF is informed by the work of the clinical physiotherapist Andry Vleeming, PhD. Vleeming is widely known for his extensive medical and research experience in functional and rehabilitative approaches to low back, pelvis, and hip biomechanics in the context of myofascial "slings" and skeletal "stacks" of the static and moving body. Formulated by his fellow clinical physiotherapists and functional movement visionaries Diane Lee and Linda-Joy Lee, the IMF pertains primarily to the centrality of the pelvis as a locomotive engine.[2] The model is represented by a feedback loop created by four overarching variables that affect robustness in relationships between the stability and mobility of the low back, pelvis, and hip complex, as seen in Figure 4.1.

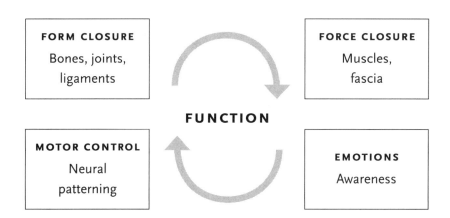

FIGURE 4.1. Integrated Model of Function

The first variable of the model is known as form closure. Form closure denotes the fit between the interacting surfaces of bones. The more contact area, the more stability in the articulation zones. Form closure refers to how we are put together skeletally, and it's a passive factor of movement in the sense that our architecture is what it is. We navigate our way along many of these joints thanks to the bony landmarks that indicate their structural terrain.

The second variable, force closure, pertains to the interactions between fascia, ligaments, muscles, and ground reaction forces. In essence, the neuromusculoskeletal system orchestrates a dynamic equilibrium between friction and compression forces to effectively transfer load through the joints. The proprioceptive senses, described earlier as the body's gravity positioning system, help initiate and mediate the give-and-take between reflexes, muscle activation patterns, and how we are bouncing around the earth, so we keep our heads above our hearts while we reach for the stars.

The third variable of the IMF is emotional awareness. At the end of the day, any division between the mind, body, heart, and spirit is an intellectual construct of convenience—or less charitably, a denial of embodied truth. Our dominant mindset directly affects our ability to maintain robust posture and movement patterns; in particular, awareness of our emotions is critical to our bodily functions. The more we try to distance ourselves from our emotions, the more we dissociate from our somatosensory state of being and functional performance.

The fourth variable spotlights motor control. Our ability to produce coordinated, well-shaped movement is dictated by the interactions between the body, its environment, and the central nervous system. "What fires together wires together" is an easy way to remember that we grow and alter neural networks as a result of learning new tricks by way of pattern repetition and revision. We add structural and functional depth to our neuromusculoskeletal command and control systems via neuroplasticity—that is, switching things up every now and then. From changing the order in a series of familiar asana to practicing movement skills on an unstable surface, we can easily add challenge factors to facilitate growth, adaptation, and resilience in our physical, spiritual, and psychoemotional comfort. A case in point: simply moving our mat from a hard floor to a carpeted one can serve as a wake-up call in Tree Pose (Vrksasana).

When we look at asana through the lenses of these elements, we can parse interactions at play anywhere in the body. Starting our inquiries at the pelvis places us at the center of the action. Large and heavy, the pelvis is the mixing bowl where natural forces such as gravity and friction combine and channel movement energy up, down, and all around the body. Sure, the head and heart get a lot of airtime. It's the pelvis, though, that is the seat of movement.

Seat of Movement: The Lumbopelvic-Hip Complex

A quick tour of the pelvis gets us in sync with our bipedal, gravity-bound selves. Our body-mapping and postural-interpreting skills will come in useful yet again. You may want to step in front of a mirror and scan the low back, pelvis, and hips from various angles with adhesive dots in place to indicate the bony landmarks. On the other hand, you may want to rely on other sensory perceptions such as feel or heft. Regardless of strategy, direct your attention to the pel-

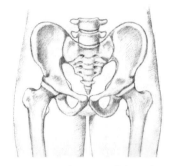

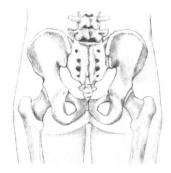

FIGURE 4.2. Close-Up of the Pelvis, Anterior View

FIGURE 4.3. Close-Up of the Pelvis, Posterior View

vis and home in on the hip axis. Refer to Figures 4.2 and 4.3, which depict close-up anterior and posterior views of the pelvis. Annotate the illustrations, labeling the various features of the pelvis to help imprint the landscape on your memory.

The hips comprise two of the largest weight-bearing joints in the body and serve as the body's primary axis of movement. These ball-and-socket joints are capable of movement in multiple planes. The hip joints move with and in relationship to the bowl-like pelvis. Their structure lends itself to power, endurance, and stability, thanks to a high degree of form and force closure. The convex head of the thigh bone fits into a deep bony socket surrounded by many layers of thick connective and muscle tissue. Well-functioning hips enable consistent and efficient responsiveness to changes in joint position, load, and force transfer. Consistency and efficiency of responsiveness (robustness) is another way to think of stability.

Above the hips, the pelvis connects to the vertebral column at L5/S1 (the lumbosacral joint) and moves relative to the low back at this transitional segment of the spine. The angle of this joint is important to visualize because it is the taproot for the lordotic curve of the low back. We intuit the acuity of this angle at L5/S1 by following the convex curve of the sacrum itself. Based on its shape, we can feel how the top of the sacrum tilts forward relative to the posterior rotation of the hip bones.

The vertebral curves are responsive to one another in a kinetic chain. When movement occurs at the lumbosacral joint, the rest of the spine will move as well. In a nutshell, move the pelvis and the axial body adjusts accordingly. The vertebral column is like an antenna tuned to a broad spectrum of postural and movement bandwidths. To experiment, tuck your tailbone while sitting or standing. You will feel your low back flatten and move into flexion. Squeeze one hip upward, into the side waist, and you will feel your low back side-bend, or flex laterally. Turn your hips and your chest and shoulders will follow.

The sacroiliac (SI) joints are also formed by the bones of the pelvis. The outer edges of the sacrum lie congruently with the ilia (hip bones), with a marked degree of surface overlap. The surfaces are knit together with layers of strong, thick ligaments spanning from the outer hips to the low back and tail, front and back. The SI joints are thus structured for load and force transfer. In other words, weight-bearing from the body above the pelvis and ground reaction forces from the earth and feet below are funneled through these articular intersections.

In addition to resistive connective tissues that sustain force closure, many muscles, large and small, act on the SI joints. There is no "sacrum-moving" muscle per se; however, the powerful glutes, pelvic floor muscles, hip abductors and rotators, and deep abdominal muscles are all at play in the force closure between the sacrum and ilia. While their range of motion is small in terms of degrees, especially when compared to what is typically available in the hips and at L5/S1, SI joint play is critical to the efficient function of the pelvis and thus the body as a whole. Without give-and-take in the SI joints, we wouldn't be able to crawl, sit down, stand up, accommodate a growing fetus, or give birth vaginally. We would also waddle like penguins, which would not lead to happy low backs, much less happy feet.

Fire Up the Belly: Core Stabilization

An undeniable principle of movement is that we must be able to stabilize in order to bear weight, transfer loads, generate power, and dissipate force. Different types of muscle activation patterns meet these many demands. Postural, or tonic, muscles hold the line in response to gravity. These slow-twitch endurance champions tend to get short and tight in response to injury, overuse, and underuse. Movement, or phasic, muscles come online in response to demand rather than gravity. These fast-twitch force mediators tend to weaken and lengthen in response to injury, overuse, and underuse.

Tonic muscles that provide postural control reside closer to the bones in the trunk. They support the vertebral column, spread compression through the intervertebral discs and joints, and maintain intra-abdominal pressure. Known as the intrinsic core stabilization system, the primary tonic muscles include deep abdominal muscles and swaths of more superficial fascia. This extensive, deeply rooted myofascial system also serves as the engine of the breath, its muscles acting as the main and accessory agonists of respiratory activity. Its fascial attachments also fuse with the inferior surface of the pericardium—the fascial sac that surrounds the heart—and the superior surface of the liver. To remark that every breath we take "massages" the heart and liver is not an overstatement given these fascial links. Heartstrings are an anatomical reality as it turns out! For more information about the tissues of this muscle group and where they lie, refer to Table 4.1.

TABLE 4.1   Intrinsic Core Stabilization System

MUSCLE/FASCIA TERM	DESCRIPTION	FUNCTIONS
Diaphragm	Parachute-like wall of muscle stretching from posterior surface of lower tip of breastbone, lower six ribs, and L1-L3; inserts into its central tendon, like a drawstring	Primary muscle of respiration; separates thoracic and abdominal cavities; helps adjust chest and belly pressure

MUSCLE/FASCIA TERM	DESCRIPTION	FUNCTIONS
Intercostals	Crisscrossed, sheetlike muscles that attach between lower border of rib above to upper border and costal cartilage of rib below	Stabilize rib cage during trunk movements; help maintain chest pressure during respiration
Internal oblique abdominals	Sheetlike muscles that run from iliac crest, inguinal ligament of groin, and thoracolumbar fascia to bottom three or four ribs and central tendinous band created by aponeurosis of abdominal wall from breastbone to pubic bone (linea alba)	Compress abdomen and hold up viscera against pull of gravity, preventing organ prolapse; contribute to lateral flexion and rotation of trunk
Multifidus muscles	Small, fingerlike muscles that span obliquely from posterior surface of sacrum near PSIS to spinous process of C2, stretching from transverse processes of one vertebra to spinous and transverse processes of vertebra above; also part of transversospinalis group	Stabilize posture and vertebral column during all movements, from L5 to C2; stabilize vertebra to vertebra; contribute to extension, rotation, and lateral flexion of vertebral column
Pelvic floor	Layers of muscles that span front to back from pubic bone to coccyx and side to side to ischial tuberosities (sitting bones)	Serves as vaginal, urethral and anal sphincters; supports intra-abdominal pressure and holds up viscera against pull of gravity; stabilizes trunk with limb movements

MUSCLE/FASCIA TERM	DESCRIPTION	FUNCTIONS
Thoracolumbar fascia	Thick, layered sheath of fascia (connective tissue) that enrobes the musculature of the back from thoracic to lumbar; integrated from aponeurosis of latissimus dorsi, quadratus lumborum, and gluteus maximus to abdominal obliques, transversus abdominis, and psoas	Stabilizes the trunk; transfers load and transmits force between shoulder and pelvic girdles
Transversospinalis group	Group of striplike muscles that run along length of vertebral column from transverse process of vertebra above to spinous process of vertebra below; includes multifidus, rotatores, and semispinalis	Stabilizes posture; contributes to proprioception; contributes to extension and rotation of vertebral column
Transversus abdominis	Sheetlike muscle that spans from iliac crest, inguinal ligament of groin, costal cartilages of lower six ribs, and thoracolumbar fascia to linea alba	Compresses abdomen and holds up viscera against pull of gravity, preventing organ prolapse; supports posture; contributes to forced exhalation as well as sneezing and coughing

Phasic muscles translate force through the joints of the trunk. Spanning from shoulder to seat, these muscles and their connective tissue partners move and stabilize the shoulders as well as adjust the depth of the rib cage. Like metaphorical marionette strings, this myofascial system manages the curves of the vertebral column and tilt of the pelvis when sitting, standing, and walking. Composed of the deep and superficial muscles of the belly, side and back waist, this team is referred to as the extrinsic core stabilization system.

These muscles maintain our center of gravity, keeping the pelvis over the thigh bones when we move our arms and legs. To learn more about these trunk movers, refer to Table 4.2.

TABLE 4.2 Extrinsic Core Stabilization System

MUSCLE/FASCIA TERM	DESCRIPTION	FUNCTIONS
Erector spinae	Group of deep, striplike muscles (also called sacrospinalis) arising from sacrum, iliac crest, ribs, and spinous and transverse processes to ribs, transverse and spinous processes, and occipital bone; includes spinalis, longissimus, and iliocostalis from spine outward to ribs	Stabilize curves of vertebral column when standing and sitting; stabilize vertebral column in relationship to pelvis during walking/running; contribute to extension and lateral flexion of trunk
External oblique abdominals	Sheetlike muscles that run from lower eight ribs to iliac crest and into linea alba via aponeurosis of abdominal wall	Compress abdomen and hold up viscera against pull of gravity, preventing organ prolapse; contribute to lateral flexion and rotation of trunk
Gluteus maximus	Thick, heavy, slablike muscle that forms the buttock; spans from outer perimeter of ilium and posterior surface of sacrum and coccyx as well as aponeurosis of erector spinae and thoracolumbar fascia to back of proximal femur and iliotibial band from tensor fascia latae	Stabilizes pelvis over thigh bones in upright posture; stabilizes lateral knee and medial long arch of foot; contributes to SI joint stability/force closure; extends and laterally rotates hip; generates power to run/jump/climb; unloads ischial tuberosities when sitting

MUSCLE/FASCIA TERM	DESCRIPTION	FUNCTIONS
Latissimus dorsi	Shawl-like muscle that covers back from spinous processes of T7-S5, back of iliac crest, lower ribs 8/9 to rib 12, and inferior angle of shoulder blade to twisted insertion into groove near head of humerus (intertubercular sulcus) beneath shoulder joint	Translates force between arms and low back/pelvis; assists with flexion and extension of low back; stabilizes shoulder blades; extends, adducts, and internally rotates arm; depresses shoulder blade; contributes to compression of chest and abdomen during coughing/sneezing and forced inhalation
Rectus abdominis	Long, flat, sheathlike muscle that helps form linea alba (tendinous band formed by entwined connective tissue of rectus abdominis, external and internal obliques, and transversus abdominis); stretches from pubic bone to bottom tip of breastbone and costal cartilages of ribs 5–7	Stabilizes pelvis during walking/running, flexes lumbar spine, and depresses rib cage

DEEPER DIVE: MIDDLE GROUND

Before any sort of physical training, asana or otherwise, (re) connect with your center by way of a neutral pelvis. Freedom to roam—as well as stay put—begins from this middle ground. Earlier, we used a doorjamb or outside wall corner to find the equanimous distribution of body weight when standing. Sometimes it's easier to identify and adjust toward well-distributed spinal curves and a well-centered pelvis with less gravity. Let's explore another route to neutral turf through Supine Pelvic Rocking. Be sure to

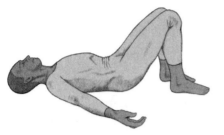
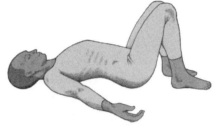

FIGURE 4.4. Posterior Tilt of the Pelvis, Side View

FIGURE 4.5. Anterior Tilt of the Pelvis, Side View

have an eye bag or washcloth nearby plus a blanket to support the head and shoulders. Refer to Figures 4.4 and 4.5, which offer side views of pelvic posterior and anterior tilts while supine.

Come down to your mat and rest on your back with your knees comfortably bent and feet hip-width apart. Rest your arms by the sides of your body. Adjust your head position until you rest on the back plate of your skull just below the occipital ridge. Your chin is on the same plane as or slightly below your forehead. Use a folded blanket to support your head, neck, and top shoulders for comfort.

Once you have the head position worked out, begin to make gentle tilting or rocking movements with your pelvis, to feel your way onto the seesaw-like ridge that runs transversely across the sacrum from left to right. This ridge indicates the most convex aspect of the sacral curve. You may need to tilt your pelvis anteriorly by way of rolling your pubic bones downward between your legs, toward the floor. You have tipped too far if you feel pinching anywhere in the low back, especially from L3/L4 to L5/S1, or if the rib points poke upward. Alternatively, you may need to roll or tuck your pelvis posteriorly to find the axis of balance on the sacrum. You have adjusted too much if you feel the top of your sacrum and low back resting or pressing on the floor—unless you are working with scoliosis, which requires a further individualized approach beyond the scope of this book.

Sense your back bottom ribs, from rib 10, and adjust the length of the waist and position of the rib cage until you feel these ribs resting on the mat—again, unless you are working with scoliosis. By resting on the sacral bony axis and back bottom ribs around rib 10/11, you are seeking the lumbosacral curve organic to your body. The head and neck will naturally follow the movements of the pelvis, so you may notice sympathetic refinements in your head position.

It will take effort to hold the pelvis and low back steady, especially when they're used to a different curve. If you are teetering on the sacral seesaw, place a small, folded cloth or a thick eye bag under your body. The prop will fill the natural space created by the bony curve from the end of the low back where it meets the sacrum to the seesaw ridge. Once you get the feel of neutral with the prop, you'll be able to find it faster.

At the Crossroads: Sling Your Weight Around

Dedicated team players, muscles work in functional units with other muscles, related fascia, and ligaments. Their dharma, or duty, is to provide the elasticity that moves bones and joints while maintaining the body's stability in relationship to gravity and the task at hand. Elasticity means that the tissues stretch in accordance with strain, along a spectrum of tolerance, and return to their original or default length after the load is removed. If tissue elasticity is overwhelmed by the work demanded of it, its structure will eventually or even immediately fail. The changed tissue shape, such as torn, ruptured, thinning, or inflamed—and remodeled signaling in the language of pain and/or limitation—reaches a tipping point where the way ahead requires a different itinerary. Hence, we assess our relationship with the adage "An ounce of prevention is worth a pound of cure." On the mat, this means we seek to develop our capacity to tolerate strain while avoiding the perils of under- and overuse.

Muscles and their attendant tissues produce and translate force through the planes in which they lie by way of contraction in response to gravity and demand. This means that movement occurs along lines of strain that spread beyond a narrowly defined structure of any muscle. Rather than being confined to a specific muscle demarcated by proximal and distal insertions, forces are transmitted within a network of tissue connections to assist in the load transfer. Known as myofascial subsystems, these networks overlap and connect with one another as needed to produce efficient, dynamic movement. If all goes well, force generation and translation is balanced with the bones and joints happily aligned. On the other hand, if tension is poorly distributed along lines of strain, the bones and joints can get out of whack and contribute to instability—with an attendant loss of power and comfort—during static or dynamic movements.

When we consider that muscles move us around, it makes infinite sense to assess our exploration of locomotion and body control starting in the seat of the pelvis. To borrow Vleeming's parlance, several anatomy slings surround the lumbopelvic-hip complex. Assuming an intact spinal cord, we essentially "walk" from the pelvis with locomotion originating from the spinal and trunk slings that run through the front, back, and sides of the body. Movement then spreads from the pelvic center of gravity through the limbs. Indeed, one of the first movement strategies employed by babies is to scoot about on their relatively heavy bottoms.

In addition to the extrinsic and intrinsic core stabilization systems, these primary anatomy slings rely on superficial and deep tissues with varying degrees of elasticity that range from stretchy to stiff. All these systems shape movement and hold our joints together as we make our way around the planet. In partnership with the core stabilization systems, these myofascial slings help control the mobility and position of the pelvis between the shoulders and legs. They support our breath as well as urinary and bowel continence. These slings also adjust tension in response to changes in terrain, both sudden and anticipated. An in-depth discussion of the anatomy slings is beyond the scope of this book;[3] however, it helps us to visualize movement coordination and control if we acquaint ourselves with their basic structural components, locations, and functions. Refer to Tables 4.3 through 4.6 for details regarding the four primary anatomy slings.

TABLE 4.3   Anterior Oblique Subsystem

The anterior oblique subsystem provides pelvic stability and movement relative to loading response from the rib cage to the foot. It functions like an abdominopelvic binder or corset and nexus of force transfer.

MUSCLE/FASCIA TERM	DESCRIPTION	FUNCTIONS
External oblique abdominals	Sheetlike muscles that run from lower eight ribs to iliac crest and into linea alba via aponeurosis of abdominal wall	Compress abdomen and hold up viscera against pull of gravity, preventing organ prolapse; contribute to lateral flexion and rotation of trunk
Internal oblique abdominals	Sheetlike muscles that run from iliac crest, inguinal ligament of groin, and thoracolumbar fascia to bottom three or four ribs and central tendinous band created by aponeurosis of abdominal wall from breastbone to pubic bone (linea alba)	Compress abdomen and hold up viscera against pull of gravity, preventing organ prolapse; contribute to lateral flexion and rotation of trunk
Rectus abdominis	Long, flat, sheathlike muscle that helps form linea alba (tendinous band formed by entwined connective tissue of rectus abdominis, external and internal obliques, and transversus abdominis); stretches from pubic bone to bottom tip of breastbone and costal cartilages of ribs 5–7	Stabilizes pelvis during walking/running, flexes lumbar spine, and depresses rib cage
Rectus femoris	Long, deep, two-headed quadriceps muscle of front thigh from ASIS and bony surface above hip socket to kneecap and onto tibia tuberosity via patellar ligament; only quadricep that crosses both hip and knee joints	Flexes hip joint; extends knee joint

MUSCLE/FASCIA TERM	DESCRIPTION	FUNCTIONS
Sartorius	Long, straplike muscle from ASIS to upper shinbone, medially near tibial tuberosity beneath kneecap	Laterally rotates and abducts hip joint; helps flex hip and knee joints; medially rotates knee joint when flexed
Conjoint tendon (anterior abdominal fascial sheath)	Thick, muscular sheath of connective tissues formed by weave of aponeurosis (broad, flat, sheetlike tendons) from internal oblique abdominals and transversus abdominis to fascial sheath of lower rectus abdominis to crest of pubic bones, along lower bony ridge of ilia up to sacrum, uniting with iliopectineal line of fascia enrobing iliacus and pectineus muscles	Reinforces lower abdominal wall; compresses abdomen and holds up viscera against pull of gravity, preventing organ prolapse
Hip external rotators	Group of striplike muscles that span from inner surface of ischium, pubic bone, and ilium to greater trochanter of femur; includes obturator internus, gemellus superior and inferior, and quadratus femoris	Help hold head of thigh bone in hip socket; laterally rotate hip joint
Tibialis anterior	Tubelike muscle that runs along front of shinbone from outer aspect at top of tibia to inner edge of foot at base of big-toe bone	Lifts up (dorsiflexes) foot; inverts foot, lifting up big-toe side of foot and turning sole of foot toward midline
Fibularis longus	Straplike muscle running down outer leg from outer aspect of fibula near knee to base of big-toe bone on inner edge of foot	Points (plantar flexes) foot; everts foot, lifting up little-toe side of foot and turning sole of foot outward

TABLE 4.4   Posterior Oblique Subsystem

The posterior oblique subsystem provides functional control and distributes compressive force during movement from the shoulder to the knee. In particular, this subsystem stabilizes the ilia, SI joints, and lumbar spine.

MUSCLE/FASCIA TERM	DESCRIPTION	FUNCTIONS
Lower trapezius	Most distal aspect of triangle-shaped shoulder and back muscle that spans from base of skull, spinous processes of C7-T12 to lateral end of collarbone, and acromion process along spine of shoulder blade	Pulls shoulder blades downward and rotates them upward
Thoracolumbar fascia	Thick, layered sheath of fascia (connective tissue) that enrobes musculature of back from thoracic to lumbar; integrated from aponeurosis of latissimus dorsi, quadratus lumborum, and gluteus maximus to abdominal obliques, transversus abdominis, and psoas	Stabilizes the trunk; transfers load, and transmits force between shoulder and pelvic girdles
Latissimus dorsi	Shawl-like muscle that covers the back from spinous processes of T7-S5, back of iliac crest, lower ribs 8/9 to rib 12, and inferior angle of shoulder blade to twisted insertion into groove near head of humerus (intertubercular sulcus) beneath shoulder joint	Translates force between arms and low back/pelvis; assists with flexion and extension of low back; stabilizes shoulder blades; extends, adducts, and internally rotates arm; depresses shoulder blades; contributes to compression of chest and abdomen during coughing/sneezing and forced inhalation

MUSCLE/FASCIA TERM	DESCRIPTION	FUNCTIONS
Gluteus maximus	Thick, heavy, slablike muscle that forms the buttock; spans from outer perimeter of ilium and posterior surface of sacrum and coccyx, as well as aponeurosis of erector spinae and thoracolumbar fascia to back of proximal femur and iliotibial band from tensor fascia latae	Stabilizes pelvis over thigh bones in upright posture; stabilizes lateral knee and medial long arch of foot; contributes to SI joint stability/force closure; extends and laterally rotates hip; generates power to run/jump/climb; unloads ischial tuberosities when sitting
Gluteus medius	Deep, scallop shell–shaped muscle from upper outer edge of ilium to upper outer surface of greater trochanter of femur	Stabilizes pelvis during weight transfer from one leg to other; abducts and internally rotates hip joint; contributes to lateral rotation of hip joint; contributes to hip flexion and extension
Iliotibial band	Long, thick tendon of fascia lata that runs from top outer edge of iliac crest, joins with aponeurosis of gluteus maximus, and attaches to outer side of proximal shinbone	Helps flex, abduct, and medially rotate hip joint, as well as stabilize outer knee

TABLE 4.5 Deep Longitudinal Subsystem

The deep longitudinal subsystem provides support and movement in the sagittal plane—during flexion and extension—from the lumbar region to the feet. It stabilizes the lumbosacral spine and pelvis from front to back. It also prevents nerve compression in the lumbar plexus.

MUSCLE/FASCIA TERM	DESCRIPTION	FUNCTIONS
Biceps femoris (long head)	Part of hamstring group that runs down back of thigh; attaches with two heads—superficial long head at ischial tuberosity (sitting bone) and deep short head at back of femur; connects to top of fibula and upper outer shinbone; group includes semimembranosus and semitendinosus, which connect to back of upper inner shinbone	Flexes knee joint and turns out lower leg during flexion; extends hip joint; stabilizes trunk at hip joint; helps connect lower limb to trunk
Sacrotuberous ligament	Broad, fanlike collagen strap from lower edge of sacrum, tailbone, ilium, and SI joint capsule to strong attachment along upper surface of sitting bone; blends with aponeurosis of gluteus maximus, long head of biceps femoris, and other sacral ligaments	Stabilizes SI joint; maintains sacral position in weight bearing, twisting, and side-bending; along with other ligaments, connects sacrum to pelvis and helps connect lower limb to trunk
Multifidus muscles	Small, fingerlike muscles that span obliquely from posterior surface of sacrum near PSIS to spinous process of C2, stretching from transverse processes of one vertebra to spinous and transverse processes of vertebra above; part of transversospinalis group	Stabilize posture and vertebral column during all movements, from L5 to C2; stabilize vertebra to vertebra; contribute to extension, rotation, and lateral flexion of vertebral column

MUSCLE/FASCIA TERM	DESCRIPTION	FUNCTIONS
Erector spinae	Group of deep, striplike muscles (also called sacrospinalis) arising from sacrum, iliac crest, ribs, and spinous and transverse processes to ribs, transverse and spinous processes, and occipital bone; includes spinalis, longissimus, and iliocostalis from spine outward to ribs	Stabilize curves of vertebral column when standing and sitting; stabilize vertebral column in relationship to pelvis during walking/running; contribute to extension and lateral flexion of trunk
Thoracolumbar fascia	Thick, layered sheath of fascia (connective tissue) that enrobes the musculature of the back from thoracic to lumbar; integrated from aponeurosis of latissimus dorsi, quadratus lumborum, and gluteus maximus to abdominal obliques, transversus abdominis, and psoas	Stabilizes the trunk; transfers load and transmits force between shoulder and pelvic girdles
Gluteus medius	Deep, scallop shell–shaped muscle from upper outer edge of ilium to upper outer surface of greater trochanter of femur	Stabilizes pelvis during weight transfer from one leg to other; abducts and internally rotates hip joint; contributes to lateral rotation of hip joint; contributes to hip flexion and extension
Gluteus minimus	Deep, scallop shell–shaped muscle from middle outer surface of ilium, just below gluteus medius, to front of greater trochanter	Helps stabilize pelvis in frontal plane; abducts and medially rotates hip joint

MUSCLE/FASCIA TERM	DESCRIPTION	FUNCTIONS
Obturators	Set of striplike muscles that span from inner surface of ischium, pubic bone, and ilium to greater trochanter of femur; part of hip external rotators group, which includes gemellus superior and inferior and quadratus femoris	Help hold head of thigh bone in hip socket; laterally rotates hip joint
Gastrocnemius	Thick-bellied, two-headed calf muscle from back of medial and lateral condyles of thigh bone to back of heel through Achilles tendon	Plantar flexes foot at ankle; helps flex knee; performs forward propulsion during walking/running
Soleus	Fish-shaped muscle beneath gastrocnemius, attached proximally from back of tibia and fibula to back of heel through Achilles tendon	Plantar flexes ankle joint; helps hold body upright by stabilizing ankle

TABLE 4.6   Lateral Stabilization Subsystem

The lateral stabilization subsystem provides support and movement in the frontal plane—side-bending, abduction, and adduction. It stabilizes the hips, pelvis, knees, and feet.

MUSCLE/FASCIA TERM	DESCRIPTION	FUNCTIONS
Gluteus medius	Deep, scallop shell–shaped muscle from upper outer edge of ilium to upper outer surface of greater trochanter of femur	Stabilizes pelvis during weight transfer from one leg to other; abducts and internally rotates hip joint; contributes to lateral rotation of hip joint; contributes to hip flexion and extension

MUSCLE/FASCIA TERM	DESCRIPTION	FUNCTIONS
Gluteus minimus	Deep, scallop shell–shaped muscle from middle outer surface of ilium, just below gluteus medius, to front of greater trochanter	Helps stabilize pelvis in frontal plane; abducts and medially rotates hip joint
Tensor fascia latae	Straplike muscle stretching from outer edge of iliac crest near ASIS to distal hip joint, merging with iliotibial band and running down to outer shinbone below knee	Helps flex, abduct, and medially rotate hip joint, as well as stabilize outer knee
Iliotibial band	Long, thick tendon of fascia lata that runs from top outer edge of iliac crest, joins with aponeurosis of gluteus maximus, and attaches to outer side of proximal shinbone	Helps flex, abduct, and medially rotate hip joint, as well as stabilize outer knee
Rectus femoris	Long, deep, two-headed quadriceps muscle of front thigh from ASIS and bony surface above hip socket to kneecap and onto tibial tuberosity via patellar ligament; only quadricep that crosses both hip and knee joints	Flexes hip joint; extends knee joint
Sartorius	Long, straplike muscle from ASIS to upper shinbone, medially near tibial tuberosity beneath kneecap	Laterally rotates and abducts hip joint; helps flex hip and knee joints; medially rotates knee joint when flexed

MUSCLE/FASCIA TERM	DESCRIPTION	FUNCTIONS
Adductors	Muscle group that includes adductor magnus, brevis, and longus; starts at front of pubic bone with magnus, also attached to sitting bone, inserts along entire length of inner thigh bone with distal tendinous strap of magnus attached to top back of medial condyle of femur	Adduct legs toward midline; stabilize hip joint; help rotate hip joint laterally and medially; extend and flex hips when moving into and out of flexion/extension
Pectineus	Short, comblike strap of muscle from upper front medial aspect of pubic bone to upper thigh bone	Adducts hip joint; helps flex hip joint
Gracilis	Long, slender, straplike muscle from lower edge of pubic bone to front of shinbone, running near tibial tuberosity medially beneath kneecap	Adducts hip joint; helps flex knee and medially rotates knee joint when flexed
Psoas major	Thick, cordlike muscle from transverse processes of L1-L5, vertebral bodies of T12-L5, and intervertebral discs of T12-L4 to lesser trochanter of femur	Flexes hip and trunk with iliacus; laterally rotates femur; maintains lumbar curve
Iliacus	Thick, cordlike muscle from front of iliac crest and anterior ligaments of L5/S1 and SI joints to lesser trochanter of femur	Flexes hip and trunk with psoas major; laterally rotates thigh
Quadratus lumborum	Thick, sheetlike muscle that spans from iliac crest and iliolumbar ligament from L5 to rib 12 and transverse processes of L1-L4	Fixes rib 12 and stabilizes diaphragm; extends lumbar spine; laterally flexes trunk; and laterally stabilizes trunk

We may intuit that our ability to get a move on is centered around the pelvis. Some of us have lived with the debility that ensues from a disordered pelvis, whether from SI joint or pelvic floor dysfunction. Regardless, we can have direct experience of the pelvic role in movement by going for a "butt walk."

Sit on the floor, if you are able, and stretch your legs out in front of you. This position is known as Staff Pose (Dandasana). Place your hands on your hips or rest them on the tops of your thighs. Without too much ado, shift your weight toward one sitting bone and roll the opposite sitting bone forward; that is, lean a bit into the left sitting bone and simultaneously pull the right one forward. Then shift your weight into the advanced sitting bone and roll the back one forward. Continue shifting your weight gently from side to side as you "walk" the sitting bones forward about twelve "paces." Then reverse direction. As you walk from your butt, notice how the same-side knee flexes as that sitting bone advances forward. Specifically, as you lean into your left side and step the right sitting bone forward, the right knee bends and drags the right foot with it. As the right sitting bone connects with the earth, the right knee straightens and the right foot advances while the complementary action of flexion arises on the left side. In other words, the legs follow the hip movements, as shown in Figure 4.6.

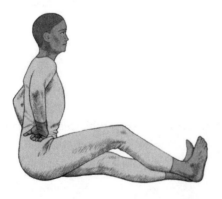

FIGURE 4.6. Staff Pose Walking

The Way Ahead: Bend without Breaking

Many of us have "issues in our tissues." Fortunately, the strength and mobility training offered by asana practice is well suited to helping our tissues—or at the very least, our attitudes toward them—adapt to bearing loads with greater tolerance. In response to strain along with gravity, the nervous system cues muscle motor units to get to work according to our wants and needs. The central nervous system also gets more efficient with practice, since it keeps track of performance successes, failures, and gaps.

Thanks to workflow management by the nervous system, muscle activation patterns turn on voluntarily (consciously) as well as automatically (reflexively). The back-and-forth between the brain and body develops our ability to tolerate strain without injury—different and/or heavier loads for longer durations and/or at a higher rate. Therein lies the key to bending without breaking: tolerance building.

Not only does the tissue-loading nature of asana hold the potential to reduce the risk of injury and other ailments, the sheer variety of poses offers myriad twists and turns to encourage a capacious neuromusculoskeletal system.[4] The more robust our ability to tolerate strain, the better our responsiveness or adaptability—and this applies to our mental and emotional health as well as our physical robustness.[5] The more adept we become at figuring out asana for ourselves, the better our quality of movement and life. Want to keep on keeping on? Judiciously challenge yourself with new tricks, old dog or no.

5

Get Organized

DEEP CORE TRAINING FOR ASANA

I have begun to think of life as a series of ripples
widening out from an original center.
—Seamus Heaney[1]

Asana emerges from the core, both physically and figuratively, of the practitioner. The gravity-inspired response code to any sort of postural or movement request is writ in the anatomical center of the body. The essence of bodily coherence resides in our ability to negotiate the weight of the pelvis whether we sit, stand, stride, or strike a pose. The limbs that get us around are tied at multiple levels and layers into the organizing axis of the vertebral column via the intrinsic and extrinsic core stabilization systems. These interwoven sheaths, straps, and strings of fascia and muscle serve as indispensable "porters" to carry the body further into safe asana practice. To get and keep a move on, we want to become travel buddies with these baggage handlers.

Consider, for example, the pose known as Standing Forward Bend. A locus of vulnerability during Standing Forward Bend practice is the zone where the hamstrings connect to the sitting bones. It's a given that forcing the body to comply with the shape of *any* pose could land us on an express train to woe. However, many of us will repeatedly, with greater or lesser degrees of subtlety, push the responsiveness of the hamstrings to "deepen" Standing Forward Bend. We absolutely must keep tissue resistance in mind, but we also need to invite more of the body into the pose.

Indeed, the path to happier—that is, intact and uninjured—hamstrings starts in the belly with core stabilization. No matter how "cooperative" our hamstrings, we simply cannot progress toward an end range of motion, and protect those back-body tendons, unless we sufficiently negotiate the weight of the body in the context of gravity. Simply put, the belly and bum are inextricably yoked together. How perfectly yogic of them!

Each of us will uncover hidden gems residing deeper in the sensory milieu of Standing Forward Bend by adding supportive resistance to its practice through the center body. Folks with more oppositional hamstrings will experience greater ease and range, especially if they lift the hands from the floor to blocks or a chair to take some of the weight out of the pose. Those of us who are able to place our hands under our feet will find enhanced stability and alertness. When we cinch the abdominal corset snugly around the trunk while moving down into the pose, the actions disperse load through the intervertebral discs and myofascial structures of the back. The resistive muscle activation helps pump the brakes so we don't topple over while folding forward and bringing the head below the plane of the heart. The myofascial laces, especially through the lumbopelvic region, act as belay ropes, pacing the descent into the somatic cave of the body. Thus, the core stabilization systems provide the time necessary for the tissues, from ligaments to nerves, to adjust to changes in loading.

As we meter our body's flow with the downward pull of gravity, we may simultaneously tap into emotions and beliefs about falling head over heels. Whether encountered in love, faith, or fear, the feelings and beliefs we hold about control, or the loss thereof, often come into view as we turn ourselves upside down. Deeper activation of the abdominal muscles, to compress or "hollow" the belly, usually reveals nooks and crannies within the gut as we settle into a static stage of the pose.

Furthermore, unearthing space within the body often channels our attention into niches within the psyche that we might have avoided or not encountered before. The light of our attention reveals more of our esoteric terrain. In other words, we enter the warm realm of Patanjali's Yoga Sutra 1:4: *Tadah drasthuh svarupe vasthanam* ("Thus the Seer is established in the light of their own radiant nature"). We tighten up the anatomical corset once again as we ascend from the pose. In addition to spinal disc and joint protection, the supportive energy we generate to lift the body back to standing reminds us that we have the capacity to rise from the ashes of sorrow, self-judgment, and suffering. Quite a journey, to say the least—and it is traversed through the core.

Travel Advisories: Proceed with Care

While core stabilization is a major component in the dynamic between gravity, posture, and movement, some of us may be working within a context of illness or injury that inhibits or interferes with this aspect of asana training. Our anatomical, energetic, and emotional realities may necessitate adjustments to if, when, and how we use the core practice series. As mentioned in earlier chapters, the gaps between wants and needs can be treacherous space.

We all have personal experience with the perils that lie between what we wish to do and what we can do safely. One of my daily mantras is taken from the warnings posted at train platforms throughout the tube, or subway system, in London: Mind the Gap. So, in the service of gap management, there are some travel advisories to heed as we proceed with mat practice.

First and foremost, be advised that strain and pain are different sensations from work and fatigue. Pain and strain feel lousy, though they serve as indispensable alerts about our relationship with the status quo. Remember, the body does not lie—and it will get our attention along a spectrum of urgency. When any action hurts— pinching, jabbing, searing, sharp, unpleasantly strong—or requires more energy than you can generate to get from point A to point B, either reduce the workload until the breath comes easily or stop immediately and regroup.

Work is a purposeful release of available energy to undertake reasonable demands or requests. Fatigue is a natural by-product of work—the expenditure of energy—and best of all, its recovery remedy is rest, a skilled practice we will come to in Chapter 7. Work and fatigue are useful sensations that help the body build robustness along a spectrum of load-tolerating capability. The core training series in this chapter and Chapter 6 are intended to move us in the direction of more efficient work and recovery.

Bulging and herniated discs in the low back region, especially at L3/L4, might make it difficult or nearly impossible to feel the "just right" of a steady, natural lumbar curve during the Tighten the Corset, Bird Dog, or Dead Bug exercises. A "just right" lumbar curve is first noted by what's absent in the lumbopelvic region: the tensions and discomforts of strain and pain. Recognition of our body's spinal curves arises with a felt awareness of the belly cavity's boundaries, inner volumes, temperature gradations, pressure variations, and movements with the breath.

Diagnosed or not, a loss of disc height may cause sufficient nerve compression to hinder the activation of the intrinsic and extrinsic core muscles. It's possible that the compression may be alleviated with diligent, judiciously paced practice within a relatively short period. Sensory and movement relief—for example, gains in trunk muscle strength; improved low back comfort; lifted mood; and greater endurance standing, walking, and sitting—may arise over the course of three to twelve weeks and thereafter require maintenance training only a couple days per week. Some of us may have more ground to cover. We may have a history of low back pain, zinging nerve surges, and atrophied trunk muscles persisting for several months, years, or perhaps decades. Thus, changes in sensation or function may take longer, such as six months or more. Continue to practice as long as the training series feels challenging yet doable and you experience perceptible effects that you enjoy.

On the other hand, disc- or joint-related nerve compression may be severe enough for long enough that the connected body part(s) feels tingly or numb. In such circumstances, neuromuscular reeducation and/or sensory recovery may prove intractably beyond the scope of self-directed movement training. If pain increases and/or function decreases after practicing the series consistently for three weeks, consider an evaluation by a licensed therapeutic movement and/or orthopedic specialist.

Individuals who have had abdominopelvic surgery, a hernia, or diastasis recti may experience a loss of sensation, scar tissue, or tissue separation that prevents or limits activation of the abdominal myofascial layers. Tissue interruptions may require specialized care and will absolutely require condition-specific body training. If you have such medical history, discuss physical yoga training with your health care provider.

Some people who have given birth vaginally or experienced other trauma to the pelvic floor may have injuries in the myofascial and sensory tissues from pubic to tailbone. If the pelvic floor activation patterns described in the Tighten the Corset and Bridge Lift exercises feel imbalanced or nonexistent from front to back or sitting bone to sitting bone, a clinical evaluation by a specialist, such as a gynecologist, proctologist, or urologist, may be helpful in identifying the nature of any disconnect, especially if you experience any urinary or bowel incontinence. You may want to discuss the use of pelvic floor training devices such as Kegel weights and physical therapy by a specialist. There are options for treatment, self-administered and otherwise. Please consider that the challenges of stress incontinence, fistula, painful sexual intercourse, and restricted movement have far-reaching, consequential health impacts. These issues are worthy of care and attention. In case you haven't heard from other sources today, *you* are worthy of care and attention.

YOGA AND SELF-CARE: QUESTIONS TO ASK YOUR DOCTOR

The documented positive effects of yoga practices are increasingly discussed in medical journals, commercial information outlets, and edutainment streams. Today, we are more likely to interact with health care providers who have some knowledge of various aspects of yoga, and physical therapists tend to be familiar with yoga-related information.

Here are five questions to discuss with your doctor, physician assistant, or nurse practitioner when seeking guidance about the appropriateness of asana for your current state of health:

1. Do you practice or have you practiced yoga? If not, do you have an opinion as to whether it might be appropriate for me?
2. What type of yoga do you recommend specifically for me?
3. What effects might I expect?
4. What are my risk factors?
5. How often do you suggest I practice?

Keep in mind, there are many styles of asana practice, ranging from gentle and slow with an emphasis on relaxation to vigorous and fast in a heated room. The yoga mat is a place of self-discovery no matter the practice style. The continuation of pain, discomfort, or ill feelings during practice is an invitation to question how we are going about our mat business rather than an indication of any sort of weakness. Instead of trying to shove a square peg into a round hole, seek expert care if you are concerned that your body is not responding to asana in a manner you enjoy.

To Thy Core Be True:
Mat Training for Postural Control

Fortified with information about how the body is structured around the lumbopelvic-hip complex to sustain and generate position and movement, we want to ensure that we are organized from our center. This is the cardinal rule of asana: no matter what we plan to do with our arms and legs, movement originates from the center of gravity in the belly space. The core training series in this chapter and the next offer skill-building and challenges to develop strength and support mobility. They train the body specifically to bear the rigors of asana, whether you practice static, slow- or fast-moving, complex or simple poses.

Work through the core training series every day for at least six weeks to plant and nourish the seeds of an integrated core before tapering off. Ideally, rely on personal progress as the measure for daily practice continuance instead of the calendar: once you can easily hold the Tighten the Corset and Plank exercises for three repetitions of sixty seconds or ten rounds of breath, then you're ready to reduce the core training to every other day and eventually once a week. Until then, practice the exercises daily. Furthermore, check in with these exercises once a month or so for the rest of your embodied life.

The most reliably accurate measure of our effort and comfort in any and every undertaking is the accessibility of our breath. Its speed and depth are unfailingly truthful metrics to gauge physical—as well as emotional, mental, and spiritual—energy expenditure. Practice each movement of the training series while breathing in and out through the nose. Not only does the nose itself serve as an air filter, heater, and humidifier but nose breathing also helps pace exertion. Any huffing and puffing through an open mouth during the asana training series means it's time to ease off and regroup.

It may take a few days to become comfortable breathing only through the nose. Like many a movement pattern, learning to breathe in and out through the nose entails building the strength and readiness for the task. Nose breathing is a learnable body-mind habit, but you need to give yourself time to ease into it. As you practice, try reminding yourself, "Now I am breathing in/out through my nose." It will become second nature over time, and you may even notice you have switched to nose breathing more frequently off the mat as well. You, or someone close to you, may notice that you are snoring less or at least more quietly. Snoring aside, nose breathing has further holistic health benefits too numerous to name here. When experiencing blocked nasal or sinus passages, experiment with breath training through narrowly parted lips. Practice inhaling and exhaling slowly and evenly. After a few rounds of parted-lips breathwork, you may even feel less pressure in the nose and head. Use the asana series to try out nose-centric breathing for yourself.

The training series will require approximately twenty to thirty minutes. Divvy it up into three- to five-minute blocks if you can't imagine adding one more thing to your daily to-do list. Sometimes it's more manageable to incorporate mini-movement breaks into the structure of your day rather than carving out a block of time.

Hopefully you have several props on hand to customize your positioning choices: one nonskid mat, two yoga blocks, one strap, two or more blankets, one bolster, one washcloth or small hand towel, and a wall. For extra options, a six- to twelve-inch inflated play or beach ball, a couple of resistance bands, and a sturdy chair are useful tools for practice. My chair preference is a folding metal chair with asana-friendly modifications, which can be ordered online from various yoga gear suppliers. Sometimes known as an Iyengar chair, it is also available from Iyengar-certified studios that offer props for sale.

In a pinch, the floor-based exercises can be adapted to standing variations at a wall—all you need to do is flip the shapes vertically. The supine and prone exercises may also be practiced on a firm bed or a sufficiently large, well-built table, for those who find the trip down to and up from the floor too far. Adapt as much as you need! Play music, set a timer, schedule a twenty-minute Corpse Pose for a later time—whatever it takes to do the work. The rewards of consistency usually arise quickly and measurably, from a more robust low back to less neck tension and improved stamina.

Deep Core Training Series: Intrinsic Core Stabilization

● ● ●

Tighten the Corset

PROPS: Nonskid mat, 2 blankets, 1 washcloth, 1 block

Sit comfortably on the mat with the props nearby. Place a blanket on the mat for extra padding and warmth, if you prefer. Ease down onto your back with your knees bent and feet placed comfortably close to your bum. Pay attention to the position of your head and neck, especially the height of the chin. A jutting chin indicates a disturbed neck curve. If your chin is higher than your forehead, place a folded blanket behind your head, neck, and upper shoulders to adjust your head position until the chin is level with or slightly below the plane of the forehead.

Now, adjust your pelvis to neutral, with the hip "points" (ASIS) and pubic bones aligned on the same plane, by tilting the tailbone downward or upward. Place a folded washcloth under the natural space formed between the sacrum and its juncture with the low back as a reminder to steady the nature archways of your low back. Wiggle some additional length out of your upper waist to relax the rib cage and rest the back bottom ribs on or nearly on the mat. Refrain from forcing the ribs down.

Place a block lengthwise between your thighs, close to the root of your body without touching. Continuously squeeze the block from the groins through the knees. Again, adjust your pelvis via small tucking or tilting actions to maintain evenness between the ASIS and pubic bones. Pull upward through your pelvic floor like you are drawing water through a straw. This action feels like you are stopping the flow of urine and any farting.

Draw the ASIS toward one another and the floating ribs toward one another by pretending you are tightening the laces of a shoe or zipping up an overstuffed suitcase. Hold the belly wall as still as possible, breathing into your side and back ribs. As you build stability, lift and hold your feet barely off the floor—without tucking your tailbone or loosening your hold on the block. Hold for 3 to 5 rounds of breath. Rest for 3 to 5 rounds of breath. Repeat three times. Gradually build to 10 rounds of breath for three repetitions.

Remember: be mindful of tendencies to push out through the belly or tuck the tailbone. From the skin through the internal organs, pull the abdominal wall down and up through the center of the belly without distorting the natural arches of your back and neck.

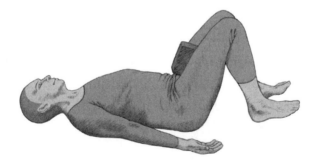

FIGURE 5.1. Tighten the Corset

Forearm Plank Pose (Chaturanga)

PROPS: Nonskid mat, 1 blanket, a wall

Ease onto the side of the body that is most comfortable for you, rest for 4 relaxed rounds of breath, then slowly sit up. Come to all fours (the quadruped position). Adjust the blanket on the mat as needed to pad your knees. Walk your body forward a bit, bend your elbows, and place your forearms on the sticky mat. Center the elbows under the shoulders. Keep your wrists straight and interlace your fingers or make fists with both hands. Press down into the little-finger sides of the hands and wrists. Visualize your shoulder blades wrapping around the side ribs like sheltering wings. Breathe steadily into the back ribs.

Walk your knees back toward the foot-end of the mat, so they are not directly under your hips. Imagine tightening a wide belt around the circumference of your belly and low back. Curl all your toes under; take more weight toward the little-toe side of your feet to encourage the legs to work without twisting the ankles. Press strongly through your heels. The straighter your legs, the more challenging the loading demands from head to feet. The intention is to move toward your knees being lifted with legs straight. Continue breathing into the back ribs, with shoulder blades steady on the midback and ribs.

From pubic bones to belly button, pull your front and side body in toward your spine. Tuck your tailbone if your bum is lifting upward and/or your low back and chest are sagging. "Stiff as a board, light as a feather," as the child's game goes. To support the weight of your head against gravity, draw your jaw inward slightly rather than letting your chin jut downward, and "reach" through the crown of your head. Push your body away from the earth. Hold this position for

3 to 10 rounds of breath, gradually increasing the duration to 16 rounds of breath. Repeat three times after resting for 4 rounds of breath between each repetition.

To earn proverbial gold stars for core stabilization, a functional benchmark is the ability to hold Plank Pose for 90 seconds (16 rounds of breath), three times with a 20-second rest interval (4 rounds of breath) between repetitions. No extra stars for anything longer than 3 minutes, since the body stops making gains useful to most of us around that mark. You may, however, enjoy working toward the benchmark and adding some stars to your practice journal.

To make the progression into a straight-leg, knees-lifted Plank Pose—first on the forearms, then with straight arms—practice with the foot-end of the mat against a wall. As you situate yourself in the starting position for the pose, walk your feet back until you can press your heels solidly into the wall. You'll need to play with wall proximity so you can straighten your knees comfortably without locking or jamming. The trick is to get the body and knees far enough from, yet close enough to, the wall that you can straighten your legs while pressing the fullness of your heels firmly into the wall with all ten toes curled under.

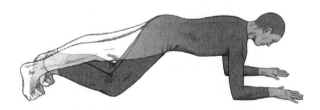

FIGURE 5.2. Forearm Plank Pose with Bent to Straight Knees

Forearm Side Plank Pose (Vasisthasana)

PROPS: Nonskid mat, 1 blanket, a wall

In this pose, the floor-side of the body is the workhorse. Lie down on the weaker side of your body first. Bend your knees to reduce strain, or keep your legs straight to increase the challenge. Keep your hips in neutral, no flexing or extending, regardless of knee position. Lift your body and place your lower forearm on the mat, with the elbow centered under the shoulder. Turn your top hip so it stacks slightly forward of the bottom one. Glue the big-toe sides of your feet together.

Remember the greater trochanter? By rolling the top hip slightly forward of the bottom, we avoid feeling an uncomfortable pressure point or hot spot. The weight of the body rests in front of the greater trochanter rather than directly on it. That said, you may want to place a folded blanket under your bottom hip for padding.

On an exhalation through the nose, lift the side body away from the floor. Your sacrum and sternum face the wall opposite you—in other words, no rotation in either the pelvis or the upper body. Keep your chin aligned with your breastbone.

If you'd like to add difficulty, reach toward the ceiling with your top arm. Alternatively, place the top-arm hand on your waist or lightly on top of your head. Pull upward through your lower side body, especially the waist. Hold your organs in your back body and resist the temptation to press outward against the abdominal wall. Stay in position for 3 to 10 rounds of breath. Perform three repetitions. Then repeat on the other side.

Notice any jaw clenching or the tongue pressing into the roof of the mouth. Relax your lips and tongue to soften your face. Smile and you might find some joy in the pose.

Ready to practice with straight legs? As in Plank Pose, try Side Plank with the soles of your feet pressed into the wall. The resistance provided by the wall may offer the oomph you need to straighten your knees while holding up your body. Eventually, experiment with straight legs and a straight supporting arm.

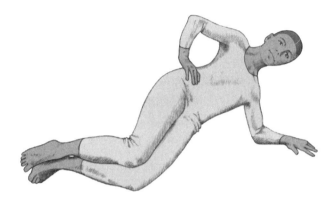

FIGURE 5.3. Forearm Side Plank Pose with Bent Knees

● ● ●

Bird Dog with Variations

PROPS: Nonskid mat, 2 blankets, 2 blocks

Pad your mat for kneeling comfort, if needed. Return to the quadruped position with knees under hips and wrists under shoulders; spread your fingers well with your weight in the base of the thumbs and index fingers. The space between the index and middle fingers points forward. Turn your upper arm bones inward until the hollows of your elbows comfortably face each other. Do not shrug your shoulders up toward your ears to achieve this movement. If your wrists get cranky, place the wide sides of the blocks on the mat under your forearms. When you support your forearms in this way, the blocks become new hands. Additionally, the blocks give you more space between your body and the mat to move your arms and legs.

Curl all ten toes under, if possible; otherwise, place a rolled blanket under the front of your ankles and press downward through the ankles into the blanket. Hold your navel lightly up toward your spine without tipping your pelvis in any direction. Imagine a full teacup balanced on your sacrum.

As you inhale, lift your left arm out to the side, slightly below shoulder height. Hold for 4 rounds of breath. Exhale and lower. Repeat with the right arm, holding for 4 rounds of breath. Repeat eight to ten times, alternating arms. One repetition equals one lift of the left arm plus one lift of the right arm. Rest as needed before proceeding with the next variation.

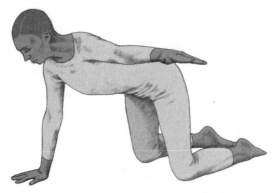

FIGURE 5.4. Bird Dog Pose with Arm Lift to Side

Return to center on all fours. When ready, inhale as you lift your left arm straight ahead, slightly below shoulder height. Resist the temptation to rotate your rib cage to achieve the shoulder flexion. You are looking for work sensations in the ab muscles right below your rib cage.

Reach gently forward through your fingertips without bending your wrist. Hold for 3 rounds of breath. Exhale and lower. Repeat with your left arm. Continue alternating the arm lifts for ten repetitions.

To increase intensity, move your knees farther back on your mat. The closer you are to a full Plank position, the more challenging it is. In fact, working toward alternating side and forward arm lifts in Plank Pose will lead to seriously useful strength gains.

If needed, prior to performing the final variation of this exercise, give your knees a reprieve by shaking out your legs or walking a few steps. When they've recovered, return to all fours. Continue to hold your navel gently yet firmly up toward your spine. Your abs are engaged so there is no laxity in the belly, yet you can breathe without force or strain.

With an inhalation, lift your left arm and right leg. Hold for 3 rounds of breath, in and out through the nose. On an exhalation, lower the contralateral pair. Then, inhale and repeat with the right arm and left leg. Hold for 3 rounds of breath, and lower on an exhalation. Continue alternating between the opposing limb pairs for eight to ten repetitions.

Remember: Hold the arm and leg at or slightly below the joint height of the shoulder and hip. It's not about how high you lift the limbs. Instead, focus on keeping your pelvis and rib cage stable, and your sacrum and breastbone facing the floor. In other words, resist the temptation to rotate your hips or shoulders to lift your limbs higher.

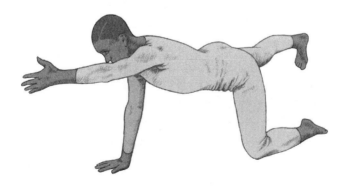

FIGURE 5.5. Bird Dog Pose with Contralateral Limb Lift

Limbs Uplifted Pose
(Urdhva Prasarita Padasana) with Variations

PROPS: Nonskid mat, 1 blanket, 1 washcloth

This pose name is more directly translated as Upward Extended Feet or Raised Stretched-Out Feet Pose. My preference is to refer to it as Limbs Uplifted Pose, since the shorthand label captures the essence of the arm/leg position without the unwieldy handle. Nomenclature reasoning revealed, let's return to the task at hand.

Lie on your back, padding the mat with a folded blanket per your preference. Place your arms along the sides of your body and bend your knees comfortably with your feet on the floor. Adjust your pelvis and rib cage to preserve the natural lumbar curve. In other words, avoid tucking your tailbone and/or thrusting upward through your ribs. Feel free to place a small, folded cloth under the top of your sacrum, per the Tighten the Corset exercise, to support the lumbopelvic arches and neutral pelvic position.

With an exhalation, draw your knees in toward your chest. Move your legs in to your body one at a time if you have wonky SI joints. Also, use your hands on the backs of your thighs to help pull your knees to your chest, if needed. The low back will flatten a little bit; however, resist the temptation to push your back down onto the mat.

On an inhalation, sweep your arms up and over your head to the floor behind you and straighten your legs until the knees are centered over the hip sockets—or center the bent knees over the hip sockets. If you keep your knees bent, support the weight of your feet by holding your shinbones parallel to the floor. Reach through your fingertips as if you could touch a wall past your head; simultaneously press through your heels as if you could stand on your feet. Hold the positions for 3 rounds of breath.

Exhale, draw your knees back to your chest, and sweep your arms down to rest alongside your body. Repeat eight times. Hold the fourth and eighth repetitions for 6 rounds of breath. Rest supine on the mat for 4 rounds of breath before proceeding with another variation of this pose or the series.

When your limbs are lifted, be sure to keep your knees directly over your hips whether your legs are straight or bent. Also, maintain a lumbar curve that is steady and comfortable—no arching or flattening. Continue channeling your low back's inner Goldilocks throughout the repetitions.

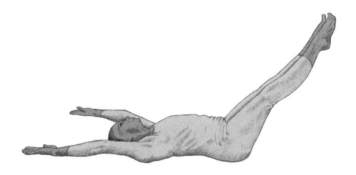

FIGURE 5.6. Limbs Uplifted Pose

To explore another layer of challenge in Limbs Uplifted Pose, add contralateral limb movements. Instead of steadying the knees directly above the hips, reach through the legs one at a time as you sweep the opposite arm overhead. You may know this exercise as Dead Bug or to borrow a phrase from Rebel Wilson's Fat Amy character in the movie *Pitch Perfect*, "horizontal running."

Despite the larger limb movements, continue to hold your pelvis and rib cage stable. Again, no rocking or twisting. To embody a smaller "bug," keep your knees bent as you lower and tap each foot lightly on the mat while reaching through the opposite arm. Practice alternating the arms and legs for 90 seconds to 3 minutes.

When you can sustain a smooth arc of movement with bent knees, progress to straight legs. First, try straightening your legs by pedal-pushing through your feet; then make it more difficult. From the starting position on your back with your arms alongside your body and thighs pulled in to your chest, straighten your legs until your knees are directly above your hips. On an inhalation, lower one straight leg toward the floor as you reach overhead through the opposite arm. On the exhalation, pull the limbs back to the starting position and repeat with the opposite pair. The straighter your leg and the closer it is to the floor, the more work necessary to stay centered in your pelvis and chest—all while inhaling and exhaling through your nose for up to 3 minutes.

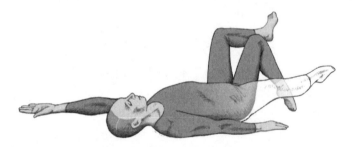

FIGURE 5.7. Dead Bug Pose with Bent to Straight Knees

● ● ●

Supine Bound Angle Pose (Baddhakonasana) with Knee Squeeze

PROPS: Nonskid mat, 1 block, 2 blankets

Roll around on the mat a bit to redistribute pressure in the back of your body. When you're ready, bend your knees and place the soles of your feet together, knees open to an easy width. Press the soles of your feet strongly into one another. Support the weight of your legs with your hands or by placing a thickly folded blanket against each outer hip and thigh. Rest your legs for a round or two of breath.

On an exhalation, press your feet firmly together and squeeze your knees slowly toward one another. Respect the range of motion and sensations in your ankles; don't try to force the knees to touch. Simply squeeze your legs toward one another without pulling the soles of your feet apart.

With the length of the inhalation, slowly "let down" or open your knees to the starting position. Use the muscle energy to support the weight of your legs and repeat the movement ten to twelve times. Keep the movement controlled and synchronized with the breath. For an added challenge, press a block between the soles of your feet—the wider the block, the more demanding for the hips and pelvic floor.

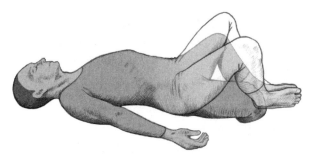

FIGURE 5.8. Supine Bound Angle Pose with Knee Squeeze

• • •

Bridge Pose (Setu Bandhasana) with Hip Lift

PROPS: Nonskid mat, 1 strap

Sit comfortably and place a snuggish strap around your ankles. (Yes, your ankles!) The strap loops across the lateral

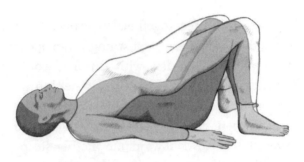

FIGURE 5.9. Bridge Pose with Hip Lift

malleoli—remember this technical term for the bony knobs
of the outer ankles?—with enough give to place the feet
hip-width apart on the mat. Make sure the strap buckle is
not pressing into your ankles, then anchor the soles of your
feet to the mat and use your arms to help ease down onto
your back.

Place your arms along the sides of your body. Wiggle some
length out of your waist, until the back bottom ribs are touching or near to touching the mat. Draw your shoulder blades
lightly toward your spine so you can feel the width of them
resting on the mat. Roll your arms away from your body, into
external rotation, so the hollows or eyes of the elbows look
toward the ceiling. Turn your forearms and palms toward
your body, into pronation, and press your palms into the mat.
Press down through your arm bones. Adjust your head so the
chin is resting just below the plane of the forehead.

Pull outward against the ankle strap without lifting your
feet off the mat. Continue pressing down through your arms
and palms. You may even find it helpful to grasp the long
edges of the mat with your hands and turn the edges under
while pulling the mat toward your feet. Think of your shoulders as another pair of feet.

On an inhalation, lift your hips to a height that engages
the glutes without tucking the tailbone. Tighten the seam of

your buttocks while pulling outward through your feet. As you exhale, slowly lower your hips to the mat. Repeat twelve times, slowly with the breath.

Rely on your glutes, partnered with your hamstrings, through the entire range of the lift. Recall that one of their primary jobs is to extend the hips, so use the "glute girdle" to create a well-shaped, controlled movement arc.

* * *

Bridge Pose (Setu Bandhasana) with Leg Lift

PROPS: Nonskid mat, 1 block

Lie on your back for Bridge Pose again, knees bent, without the ankle strap. Place your feet hip-width apart with your heels comfortably close to your bum. Adjust your feet so that the tips of the second toes point directly forward. Root the soles of your feet onto the mat. Place your arms along the sides of your body.

Draw comfortable length through your waist, until the back bottom ribs are touching or near to touching the mat. Retract your shoulder blades lightly toward your spine so you feel stable through the breadth of your shoulders. Rotate your upper arms outward and simultaneously turn your forearms and hands inward. Press down through your arms. Adjust your head so the chin is resting just below the plane of the forehead.

Pull outward through your heels without lifting your feet off the mat or twisting your ankles. Continue pressing down through your arm bones. To add support, firmly grab the long edges of the mat and pull down toward your feet.

On an inhalation, lift your hips to a sustainable height. The glutes should work strongly without clenching, and the pelvis should feel supported and stable. On an exhalation, lift your right foot off the mat and squeeze your knee in toward your chest. On an inhalation, lower your right foot back to the mat. With the next exhalation, lift your left foot off the mat and squeeze your left knee in to your chest. With the next inhalation, lower your left foot to the mat. This is one repetition. Keep your hips lifted, if you can. Otherwise, exhale and lower your hips to the mat between each repetition—or between each leg lift, if needed.

The goal is to perform twelve slow, steady repetitions while holding the Bridge Pose. If this seems like an unreasonable idea, consider that slow and steady begets slow and steady. In other words, take an incremental approach over six to twelve weeks. Especially if you have a history of low back or SI joint pain, place a block under the center of your sacrum, to lift and support the weight of your pelvis. Then try lifting your feet off the floor just a bit. Gradually add height to the leg lift and pelvis. Eventually, if you're able, try this exercise without the block support.

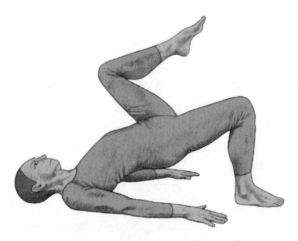

FIGURE 5.10. Bridge Pose with Leg Lift

Supported Corpse Pose (Savasana)

PROPS: 3 to 4 blankets, 1 bolster or pillow,
1 large towel, and lightweight eye cover

Welcome to Corpse Pose! This is an official rest stop. Rest is an integral part of any journey. It allows us to check in with ourselves while we replenish our energy, inventory our resources, review how far we've come, and plan for the road ahead.

Rest helps the brain and body process and retain new information and skills. Sufficient rest is a major component of learning, especially when it comes to memory consolidation and sensory integration. There is a fast-growing bank of research that definitively demonstrates mind-body interventions like yoga—especially when practice combines active movement with directed breath and attentional focus—provide a wide range of benefits, including improvements in motor control, emotional regulation, and attention.[2]

Want to support learning gains and executive function as well as self-regulation? Take a 20-minute "nap" with Supported Corpse Pose. If a 20-minute break is but a dream, spend 5 to 10 minutes in a comfortable seated position with your attention directed to the sensations of the breath.

Use one or two folded blankets to support your head, neck, and shoulders. Place a bolster, pillow, or rolled blanket behind your knees, and a rolled blanket behind your ankles. Once settled, wrap a folded blanket or large towel around your hips like a wide belt. Then cover your body from chin to toe with a blanket, shield your eyes with a light cloth or eye bag, and marinate for 20 to 45 minutes. Need something to "do" in this pose? Focus your attention on the sensations of the breath as it moves in and out of your body via your nose or lightly parted lips. Whenever you notice your mind has drifted, redirect your attention to the feelings, inner colors and sounds, depth and rhythms of body breathing.

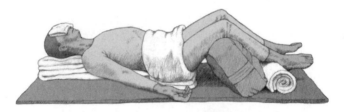

FIGURE 5.11. Supported Corpse Pose

Ab Aware, Asana Prepared

We can save ourselves a lot of soreness and outright suffering, bodily and emotional, in all manner of movement, postural, and task demands by training our intrinsic core stabilization system as a precursor to progression. While playing with "bug" movements may not seem all that dramatic or even "yogic," these are essential body skills that enable us to successfully go further into our own asana practice. The improvements in somatosensory and motor control competencies, combined with tandem gains in attention and focus, provide a resilient foundation to investigate the wide gamut of asana as well as to carry a backpack, shovel snow, and sit comfortably. The physical strength and stability gains are integral to folding forward, standing on one leg, and transitioning from one pose to the next.

Imagine walking or signing in to a new in-person or online asana class—or embarking on a walking-centric excursion—knowing you have the body awareness and physical skills to safely and satisfyingly move from standing to supine and anywhere in between in the context of your own physicality. Core stabilization gets us moving, and motion control keeps us centered while we're at it.

6

Stay Centered

MOTION CONTROL TRAINING FOR ASANA

Stay in the center, and you will be ready
to move in any direction.
—Alan Watts[1]

A well-conditioned core is a responsive one, primed and prepared to hold us together however we position ourselves to meet the moment. The previous series focused on exercises that help us tune in to and sync up the deeper myofascial tissues of the center body (the intrinsic core stabilization system). Since a gradual approach best serves integration, we start our asana skill-building close to the earth. Learning to stabilize in floor-based positions like Limbs Uplifted Pose and Bridge Pose feeds the neuromusculoskeletal roots of more dynamic movement.

The more connections we make with our inner stabilization system, the easier it becomes to toe the postural line in response to gravity. And the steadier we are in keeping our center, the more able we are to control motion reliably across a wider spectrum of demand. Since we want to follow the pathways of natural movement, we need to train the extroverted, on-call muscles that shape the forces responsible for the body's course. Thus, in this chapter, we turn our attention to the extrinsic core stabilization system.

The extrinsic core stabilization system, or outer core, helps to create smooth, controlled movement. Phasic muscles, the myofascial alchemists of the outer core, disperse body forces to adjust range, direction, and speed of motion. In a sense, the outer core protects us from our own ambition by tempering our pace and extent of loading. A demand-responsive system rather than a gravity-driven one like the deep core, the phasic muscles will work against the prime movers of a given movement arc to prevent them from overperforming and disrupting balance. They will also work in tandem with postural muscles to dial in a specific movement pattern or body orientation. These movement shapers will also tighten up to compensate for functional weaknesses.

There's a bias in the yoga world to confront "tight" tissues with stretching. Got sciatica? Do Pigeon Pose (Kapotasana). Low back feel achy and stiff? Do Child's Pose (Balasana). However, stretching muscles that are already overworking to distribute the costs of movement is counterproductive to creating healthy, durable change. Pigeon Pose may provide temporary relief to tight hips, but its time in the spotlight comes much later in the body-training journey. Introduced too early and aggressively, stretching can overwhelm tightness that is tissue- and joint-protective. Too often we focus on so-called flexibility in asana at the expense of motion control.

We need to strengthen the stabilizing and force-shaping systems of the core before we even attempt to change "tightness" anywhere in the body. That's the reality, yoga-curious friends. To stretch or gain flexibility, much less find relief, we must get and stay organized from our center so we can make our way out to and back from our personal edges. You don't climb a mountain unless you are certain you can make it back down.

Powering up the core stabilization systems allows us to follow movement pathways that lead in the direction of Triangle Pose and series like Sun Salutation (Surya Namaskar). Thus, we practice training exercises that help us safely hinge, lunge, pull, push, rotate, squat, and step. Refer to Tables 4.1 and 4.2 for a refresher on the myofascial players in the intrinsic and extrinsic core stabilization systems.

Mat Training Reminders: Buckle In and Breathe

The extrinsic core stabilization training series includes complex movements that build balance and strength. It is intended to challenge how well we stand on one leg, move our arms and legs in relation to one another, and swing our weight around. Once again, it is time to enliven that inner Goldilocks. Let your felt sense of steadiness be the arbiter of how far and fast to practice each exercise. Slow and steady wins the race, to combine fables, especially if you have a history of bulging and/or herniated discs, SI joint dysfunction, traumatic brain injury, or vertigo.

A headlong rush into the movements will defeat the intended purpose of the training: to cultivate motion control in such a way that movement feels more organic and intelligent. By its very nature, growing the skills to unlock ease in the body, breath, and mind is a prolonged process. Though it may feel like a commodity that's in short supply, time is firmly on your side. This type of functional movement training yields noticeable, sometimes speedy gains in balance, coordination, and even grace. However, those gains are sustainable only when practice is gentle and consistent. We stay on the path toward asana at the pace of the body, not the mind. So keep your eye on the prize and buckle in for the long haul.

Since we are learning to feel how our bodies move, breath awareness is no less important during this practice series. Indeed, it is the ultimate body sense that gauges our state of being. Strain in the breath indicates strain in the body, and it needs to be attended to immediately. If your ability to comfortably inhale or exhale is impinged, reduce the amplitude of the movements by way of the specified props and support for each exercise. Tools for practice, like resistance bands and blocks, invite us to tailor the size, shape, and degree of strain. By fitting the poses to the individual person, we create the conditions that allow each of us to breathe at our body's own rhythm and figure out what feels natural, safe, sweet, and steady. With the breath as our Beatrice, we return home to the joyful, unerring wisdom of the body.

Motion Control Training Series: Extrinsic Core Stabilization

● ● ●

Wall-Supported Standing Side Bend (Indudalasana)

PROPS: Nonskid mat, 1 strap, 1 block, a wall

With strap and block in hand, stand in Mountain Pose with the right side of your body near a wall. The farther you stand from the wall, the more intense the stretch. Start about a block-length from the wall, then adjust the distance accordingly. Plant your feet hip-width apart, with the space between the second and third toes pointing forward, and place a block between your upper thighs, close to the root of your body without touching. Roll your thighs slightly inward to engage your legs and calibrate your pelvis into steady neutral. Secure the strap in a loop and place it around your wrists like a big rubber band. Adjust the size of the loop so your hands are about shoulder-width apart. Lightly clench your fists and keep your wrists straight.

On an inhalation, sweep your arms over your head while pulling outward on the strap. On an exhalation, bend sideways toward the wall and rest your right knuckles against it. Keep rolling your legs gently yet insistently inward against the block while dragging your rib cage off your waist. Continue sliding your knuckles up the wall, strap taut, reaching up and over as if you could push through the wall. Turn your breastbone upward to rotate your rib cage slightly. This action will help distribute the side bend through the trunk.

Breathe into the left side of your rib cage, spreading the ribs. Hold for 4 to 6 rounds of breath. With an inhalation, pull your body slowly back to center. Lower your arms to the starting position with an exhalation. Reside in Mountain Pose for 3 rounds of breath before proceeding to the other side.

Perform this pose to stretch the left side first, then the right, then the left side again. If you are left-handed, try swapping the order. Practice Standing Side Bend as often as you like, especially after a long spell of sitting, to relieve neck, shoulder, and midback fatigue as well as to rebalance the sides of the body. Be sure to support the weight of your rib cage throughout the entirety of the pose. Reach upward through the little-finger sides of your arms continuously, without squeezing your head.

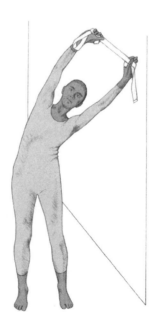

FIGURE 6.1. Wall-Supported Standing Side Bend

Wall-Supported Standing Twist (Marichyasana)

PROPS: Nonskid mat, 2 blocks, a wall

Stand in Mountain Pose approximately 8 to 10 inches from the wall (slightly less than forearm length) with the right side of your body parallel to the wall. Place a block on the floor in front of your right foot. How confidently you can balance on one leg determines the height and number of blocks you use to lift your foot. The higher the foot, the more challenging it is to balance. Keep in mind your ability to resist the downward pull of gravity when selecting the height of the foot support.

Place your right hand on the wall with the fingertips slightly below the top of your right shoulder. Step your right foot onto the block support and press downward from hip to heel. On an exhalation, keeping your pelvis stable and facing forward, turn your upper body toward the wall. Move your right hand to the right as necessary. Place your left hand on the wall slightly below shoulder height, and press into the wall through the left arm. Think of those frontal plane-oriented facet joints from the top of the T_{12} vertebra upward. Turn your body from the bottom of your rib cage like you are steering a bicycle around a curve. Pull your belly button back and in toward your spine, with the left lung turning to the right. Hold the Standing Twist for 4 to 6 rounds of breath.

On an exhalation, unwind back to center from the bottom of the rib cage, with your chin centered and riding along with your breastbone. Step your foot down and abide in Mountain Pose for 3 rounds of breath. Turn around and perform on the other side. To repeat the Standing Twist, experiment with different patterns, such as left-right-left or left-left-left-right-right-right.

If you have strong flamingo skills, place your right foot on the seat of a metal folding chair. No matter the height of the foot support, resist hitching the same-side hip to lift and hold the foot position. Instead, work to pull the wall-side foot up and onto the blocks or chair seat by using the hip flexors and lower abdominal muscles. If you are unable to lift your foot onto the support without pulling up through your outer hip, work with both feet on the floor for a couple of weeks. Then take another foray into the lifted-foot variation.

Lots of folks mimic owls and overwork the head and neck rotation. Basically, we give ourselves the illusion of the full body twist by leading with the head. Avoid this shiny fishhook of *maya* ("illusion") by keeping your chin aligned with your breastbone throughout the twist, and move slowly and deliberately.

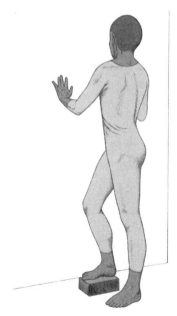

FIGURE 6.2. Wall-Supported Standing Twist

Revolved Warrior I (Parivrtta Virabhadrasana I) with Resistance Band

PROPS: Nonskid mat, 1 resistance band

This is a complex vinyasa that asks a lot of the body. By adding the element of resistive rotation to the big lunge movement—and doing so when stepping backward into the lunge position—all the core stabilizers get to come to the movement party. To ensure everyone plays well together, you may want to practice this vinyasa a couple of times without the resistance band. When you do add the band, err on the side of less resistance, and take your time switching up to tighter bands.

Stand near the front end of the mat in Mountain Pose with the resistance band in hand, feet hip-width apart. Grasp the ends of the band and inhale as you bring your hands to a loose Prayerful Mudra at the chest. With an inhalation, take a reasonably long step backward with your right leg, planting the right foot directly behind the right hip, and straighten your legs. The toes of your front foot will turn out slightly—about a big-toe width for most of us. Now, look at your back foot. The toes should point almost directly forward. Have a Goldilocks moment and adjust the turnout of each foot in increments for steadiness. It's particularly important to press firmly down through the little-toe side of the back foot to better anchor the body and avoid rolling into the inner foot and knee of the back leg.

Once grounded in your feet and legs, exhale and press your body down into a left-leg lunge from hip to knee to ankle. Tell the outer hip and upper thigh muscles to pull your body down into the lunge. The front knee tracks toward the second toe on the front foot. It's safe for the knee to flex forward of the ankle and creep toward the tips of the

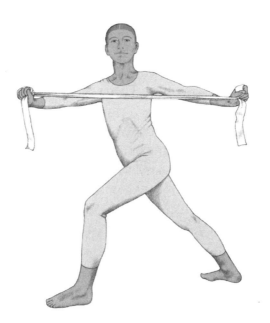

FIGURE 6.3. Revolved Warrior I Pose with Resistance Band

toes, or even a little past. It happens with every step as we climb the stairs. Simply keep your heels grounded and your feet steady.

Your pelvis should be facing toward the front of the room without force or strain. If the lumbosacral region feels pinched or crowded, widen your stance from left to right by stepping the back (right) leg to the right. By shifting the back foot laterally, we give ourselves more room to move. Engage the back leg as an anchor for the lunge: press down through the back heel, forward through the calf muscles, and backward through the thigh bone. Hold your body as vertically as comfortable, balancing the chest cavity over your belly and your head over your chest.

With the next exhalation, turn your entire torso to the left, toward the front leg, while pulling the resistance band taut like an archer drawing a bowstring. Stay here for 3 rounds of breath. With an inhalation, slowly turn back to center while bringing your hands together at the chest and straightening your front leg. Repeat four times, slowly and deliberately. With an exhalation, step the back leg up to Mountain Pose and rest for 3 rounds of breath. Then change sides and perform four repetitions.

Once you feel confident with the movements, speed up and step back directly into the lunge position while pulling on the resistance band. Also try alternating between the sides at a breath-friendly pace. Allow the breath to meter your effort and inform you when exertion exceeds capacity. We are not only building physical skills for asana. We are also building observational and empathetic skills to cultivate our attentional focus and awareness on and off the mat.

● ● ●

Wall-Supported Downward-Facing Dog Pose (Adho Mukha Svanasana)

PROPS: Nonskid mat, a wall

Stand in Mountain Pose facing the wall. Place your hands comfortably on the wall at shoulder height, with the index fingers pointing up toward the ceiling. Step away from the wall and begin to fold at your hips. As you fold along the hip axis, walk your hands down the wall and step your feet back so your knees and ankles align under your hips and your arms are straight. Imagine your body squaring a box with the wall.

The closer the body comes to a ninety-degree angle at the hip joints, the stronger the desire of the low back to flex or round and the more need we have for trunk support. You may notice your abdominals supporting your flattened low back, working against the downward pull of gravity and body weight. Encourage the muscles to hold the line by pulling the abdominal wall in and up from your pubic bones to your rib cage. Imagine pulling and squishing your internal organs up against the front (anterior) spine.

Inhale, press your hands into the wall, and slide your shoulder blades toward the base of your skull. Exhale and pull your shoulder blades down toward your waist without losing contact with the wall. Repeat the shoulder blade slides six times. Then walk your body toward and up the wall with an inhalation, and return to Mountain Pose.

Instead of rounding the back to "square the box," adjust the depth of the forward bend and hand height on the wall to activate the abdominals. Our intention is to improve transitional strength, such as when moving into and out of forward bends. Skipping the work by flexing at T12/L1, L3/L4, and/or L5/S1 increases the odds that we will part ways with low back comfort and function on very poor terms. In other words, rounding the back—including any "roll-up-one-vertebra-at-a-time" business—sets up an ugly fight with gravity that the low back will lose. Keep tugging the strings of the body's many-layered corset to stabilize your spine as you fold and straighten from the axis of the hips.

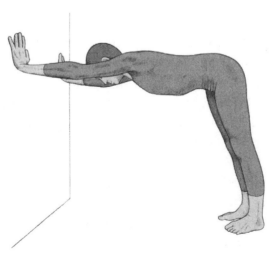

FIGURE 6.4. Wall-Supported Downward-Facing Dog

Tree Pose (Vrksasana) with Variations

PROPS: Nonskid mat, a wall

Return to Mountain Pose, standing near the wall. You may want to face, align the side of your body with, or stand with your back to the wall. Regardless of position, the wall is a support, not a bed, so avoid leaning against it.

Check your foot placement and adjust the width until your legs feel solid under your body. For most of us, the feet are most naturally placed one to two fist-widths apart. When you're ready, on the length of an inhalation, lift both heels and shift your weight into the balls of your feet without wobbling through your ankles or clenching your toes. As you exhale, slowly lower your heels. Place your hands or fingertips on the wall for support as you raise and lower your heels. If your foot and ankle control is solid, sweep your arms up over your head along with the heel raise. Coordinate the heel raise and arm lift with the length of each inhalation and exhalation. Also, pace the heel and arm raises to reach the apex of each at the same moment. Practice six to eight times, then stand quietly in Mountain Pose for 3 rounds of breath.

Once you're steady, prepare to shift all your weight into one leg based on your dominant side. To encourage learning, we will first stand on the leg of the nondominant side—if you're left-handed, begin with standing on the right leg and vice versa. Since most folks are right-handed, note that the instructions commence from the left side. Again, practice according to your individual needs.

Place your hands on your hips and turn the toes of your left foot out, no more than a big-toe width. For added stability, place the fingertips or palms of your hands on the wall. Shift some of your body's weight into your left leg. Instead of locking your standing-leg knee into a straight position, press down into the front edge of the heel and across the ball of the foot without clenching the toes. Squeeze the calf muscles of the standing leg inward, against the back of the shinbone, like you are about to lift your heel. In response to the calf action, the muscles of the thigh will turn on to stabilize the weight-bearing knee. Since that standing leg represents a tree trunk, embrace the resilient solidity of the fully engaged leg.

Continue to shift your weight into your left leg, and as you exhale, draw your right knee up toward your chest as high as possible without rounding your back. Hold your right leg up for 3 rounds of slow, steady breath, as if frozen in a marching position. Then, on an exhalation, lower your right foot to the mat. Repeat twice more, with a full round of breath between each repetition. If you feel up to the task, raise and lower your right knee and left arm at the same leisurely pace, in harmony with the breath. Repeat with each opposing pair three times.

Return to Mountain Pose and notice how you feel. Take 3 rounds of breath, then lift your right knee out to the side, toward your right shoulder, without crunching into the side waist or leaning to the left. Without disturbing your balance, press the sole of your right foot against the inner calf or thigh of your left leg on its own power, at an unforced height. Remember, we are focused on developing motion control in Tree Pose rather than spelunking into some of the more eso-teric ideas about asana right now. Please trust that exploring the effects of energy seals on pranic flows will come to bear once we consistently keep our center. To that end, don't be shy about placing that lifted foot on a block until you feel solid in the standing leg. You might also try resting the outer knee of the lifted leg, instead of your hands, against the wall.

Hold your right leg up for 3 rounds of breath, then lower your foot to the mat with an inhalation. Repeat twice more, with a full round of breath between each repetition. Then switch sides and repeat the series while standing on the opposite leg.

Once you're able to practice each variation smoothly, add arm movements. As you lift the leg, reach for the sky by sweeping your arms out and up. Your arms represent the branches of a tree, so let them grow. Visualize the wingtips of the shoulder blades pulling away from one another and gliding upward along the ribs, with the arm bones along for the ride. Feel your shoulder sockets orient in the same direction as your arm bones, and stretch upward through the little-finger sides of your arms. If you feel any pinching in your shoulders and/or the base of your neck, widen the space between your arms. Spread your crown, opening more of your branches to the sun's radiance.

As you practice each variation of Tree Pose, notice differences in balance between the standing and lifted legs. Most of us feel more stable on one side versus the other. You've probably determined by now that the roots are less secure when standing on your nondominant leg, which is exactly why we start on that leg in the first place.

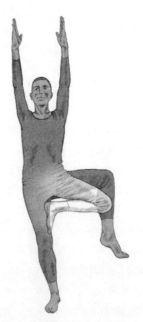

FIGURE 6.5. Tree Pose with Variations

Warrior III Pose (Virabhadrasana III) with Variations

PROPS: Nonskid mat, a sturdy chair, 1 to 6 blocks

We are about to embark on a big movement arc in this dynamic variation of Warrior III, which is also a type of single-leg deadlift. You may want a sturdy chair to hold on to. Otherwise, practice with your arms down by the sides of your body.

Reestablish Mountain Pose at the center of the mat. Shift your weight into your nondominant leg—for now, the left leg. Inhale slowly, steadily, and evenly. With the start of the next exhalation, fold forward at the standing-leg hip while simultaneously lifting the opposite leg to hip-height behind you. Resist any inclination to kick the leg back and up or twist your hips to lift the leg higher.

Focus on breathing into your side ribs and pulling the belly energy in through your navel. Think about drawing your abdominopelvic organs up into your body so there's no laxity through the belly walls. Reach through your fingertips, as if you could touch the wall behind you. Your arms should be active without squeezing into the side ribs. Hold Warrior III for 1 to 3 rounds of breaths. Then, with an inhalation, pull your body up and lower the lifted leg to the mat. Abide in Mountain Pose for 1 complete round of breath. Then repeat Warrior III twice more on your nondominant side before switching legs.

After you can smoothly practice three repetitions on each leg, it's time to level up. If you trust your balance, pick up a block and hold it comfortably between your hands at the center of your chest. Proceed into Warrior III and tap the end of the block on the mat under your chest. As you return to Mountain Pose, carry the block back up to the heart center.

Once you can practice the single-block pickup with confidence, try a more rigorous variation with more blocks. Arrange a semicircle of 2 to 6 blocks around the end of the mat. If you don't have that many blocks, substitute beanbags or another set of easy-to-handle items.

Begin in Mountain Pose. Exhale and move into Warrior III on your nondominant side, then pick up the block farthest to the left. Inhale and rise with the block in hand, then exhale into Warrior III and lower the first block back to its starting position. Inhale and rise to Mountain Pose. Repeat with each block, lifting and lowering them from left to right and right to left. Then, after a sojourn in Mountain Pose, proceed to the second side.

When you feel like you can ride the entire movement wave, practice the block pickups without lowering the lifted back foot to the mat between each repetition. Move into and out of Warrior III by way of Tree Pose with the lifted leg to the front. As you rise from Warrior III with a block in hand,

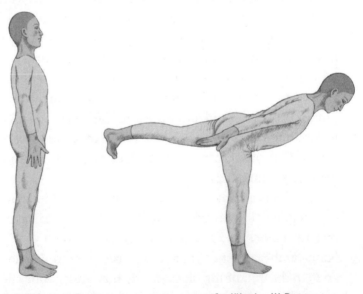

FIGURE 6.6. Mountain Pose   FIGURE 6.7. Warrior III Pose

sweep and squeeze the back leg forward and up toward your chest, without rounding your low back. Then, as you lower the block back to the mat, sweep and straighten your lifted leg back and up into Warrior III. Work through the entire semicircle—left to right, right to left—without touching the mat with the foot of the moving leg. Now perform the same series on the other side. This variation is intense, so work toward it slowly—and spare yourself any self-recrimination if it doesn't make sense for any number of reasons or concerns.

● ● ●

Derotational Forearm Plank Pose (Chaturanga) with Uneven Elbows

PROPS: Nonskid mat, 2 blankets, a wall

Transition to all fours. Place your forearms on the mat under your shoulders. Adjust your knees to correspond with a manageable load. Use a folded blanket to pad your knees, if you prefer. Remember, the more directly under the hips the knees are placed, the easier this pose will feel. Start with less load, and gradually increase intensity over time.

Curl all ten toes under and press firmly through your heels. Use a rolled blanket under the front of your ankles and press down into the blanket to compensate for unwilling toes, as needed. For more intensity, set your knees back from your hips and press through your heels until your knees lift into the straight-leg Forearm Plank. Maintain a neutral pelvis, if you can; otherwise, tuck your tailbone for bigger muscle engagement and more support.

On an inhalation, slide your left elbow about 2 inches forward of the right. We are using asymmetry in limb position to work deeply into the left-side body. Press down through your forearms while pulling up through the front of your body and pressing back through your heels. Do not let your spine get sucked into your body—no sagging! Hold the position with the uneven elbows for 6 to 10 rounds of breath.

On an exhalation, align your elbows and lower the knees. Walk your knees forward, as needed, to rest for 3 rounds of breath. When you're ready, reposition your knees and repeat with your right elbow forward. Perform three sets, holding each asymmetrical elbow position for up to 10 rounds of breath with a 3-breath break between sides: left-right, rest, left-right, rest, left-right, rest. Also, try the Derotational Plank from right to left. Notice the differences that arise when you swap the order of elbow placement.

This variation of Plank Pose enables you to have an especially robust conversation with your obliques. Reduce the time spent in the pose as needed and gradually add time as your tolerance builds. The inclination to cheat the clock may be hard to quell. For the duration of each pose, keep your hips on the same plane as your shoulders. If your bum lifts higher than your upper back, then bring your knees down to the mat. Again, reduce load rather than trying to pull yourself out of the pose. When you're able to hold for 10 rounds of nose breathing, practice without resting between the sides.

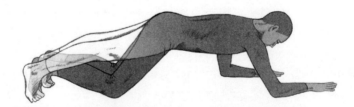

FIGURE 6.8. Derotational Forearm Plank Pose
with Uneven Elbows and Bent to Straight Legs

Cat-Cow Pose (Marjaryasana-Bitilasana)

PROPS: Nonskid mat, 2 blankets, 2 blocks

Return to all fours, with your knees and ankles supported with blankets, if desired. Set your hands shoulder-width apart, with the back of the wrists even with the top of your shoulders. The space between the index and middle fingers should point forward, and the eyes of the elbows look toward one another. Support the weight of your head and body through an alert, at-the-ready belly. Your sitting bones should neither roll under nor tilt upward. Inhale into the skin of your back and exhale without softening your body downward.

With a slow, steady exhalation, roll your sitting bones under, strongly pull your belly in and up from the pubic bones to the ribs, and round your upper back. Let your head drape downward. Take a round of breath in the "startled cat" position.

With a slow, steady inhalation, roll your sitting bones up and stretch the front of your body, from the pubic bones through the top of your head. Reach upward through your crown, stretching the front of your throat while supporting the weight of your head. Take a round of breath in the "happy cow" position.

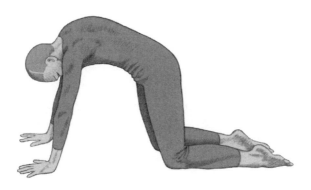

Figure 6.9. Cat Pose

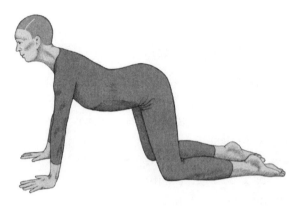

FIGURE 6.10. Cow Pose

Alternate between Cat and Cow Pose for as long as you like, coordinating the movements with each exhalation and inhalation. Move attentively and deliberately. Pay particular attention to the sensations and exertions of your belly.

● ◉ ◉

Supported Corpse Pose (Savasana)

PROPS: Nonskid mat, 3 or more blankets, 1 large towel,
1 bolster, and a lightweight eye cover

Whether you think you need to or not—and trust yourself, you need to—take a load off and settle into a supported position of rest. If you feel resistant to a fifteen-minute interlude of peace and quiet, do it anyway. Ignore the chatter in your head about how busy you are, how little time there is, how much other people are counting on you and only you. You know you're tired. How in the world does staying tired make it easier to learn or do anything? How does exhaustion help us get here, there, or somewhere any faster?

Short answer: tiredness begets tiredness. On the other hand, rest begets recovery. And recovery begets energy and agency. So stop and stay awhile in Corpse Pose. Per the guidance in the previous chapter, use nest-making accoutrements likes blankets, bolsters, pillows, and towels to create comfort for yourself. Rest quietly for at least 15 minutes, but 20 to 40 minutes if possible.

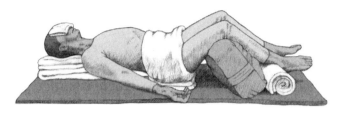

FIGURE 6.11. Supported Corpse Pose

Abiding in Ease

While we are deciphering the codes between anatomy, posture, and movement, we are also plumbing the depths of our beliefs, the direction of our thoughts, and our capacities for agency. You know for yourself that your mindset and heart song shift along with your muscles, tendons, ligaments, and joints in response to instinctual movement. As we more readily recognize how to hold the bodily center, we unleash insights into other forces—be they psychological, social, spiritual, or superstitious—that sustain, constrain, and antagonize us. Fortunately, there are more yoga practices to help us process the revelations—and (r)evolutions—that we are storing in our bodies.

7

Feel Refreshed

REST, REFLECT, AND REGROUP

Like an ability or a muscle, hearing your inner wisdom is
strengthened by doing it.
—Robert H. Gass[1]

It takes many rounds of trial and error to figure out how asana
emerges from our known and unknown spaces. To locate and navigate these inner reaches, we build our mat skills with the core training series in the previous two chapters and related investigations
such as body mapping in Chapter 2. However, mat skills like anatomical familiarity and core stabilization are just aspects of asana
practice, and asana is so much more than outcome-oriented exercise. It engages intersecting skills of the body, brain, mind, heart,
and spirit. Even if our overarching motivation for stepping on the
mat is to touch our toes in Standing Forward Bend, we automatically and simultaneously build our powers of attention, discern-
ment, and self-regulation.

Recall that yoga is a holistic system of thought, word, and deed for truthful living and inner contentment explained as the Eight Limbs in Patanjali's Yoga Sutras. Asana itself is only one of the Eight Limbs. Moreover, each of the limbs is dependent on the others to nurture awareness and peace in all levels of our being, spanning from the individual to the universal.

By now we have experienced the aftereffects of core stabilization training: feelings of calm clear-headedness and felt presence of the body, that sense of density combined with spaciousness recognized immediately as organic and natural while sporting a déjà vu quality. It becomes easier to feel this embodied intuitiveness the more we practice things like asana. The more often we connect with the sensations and emotions alive in our bodies, hearts, and minds, the more trust we create within ourselves.

Fortunately, the other limbs of yoga practice also nourish this trust in our inner wisdom and vision for living peaceably in the here and now. A short summary of yogic philosophy about the causes of suffering and nature of being, along with some contemporary science, shines a light on the benefits of adding the practices detailed later in the chapter to our daily lives. After all, we've already stepped onto the mat, so we might as well explore more rarefied terrain.

Lies, Layers, and Limbs

Despite the many (r)evolutions since the Yoga Sutras were first shared, the essential trials and tribulations that feed the roots of human suffering continue to be reflected in modern living. Plenty of analyses, from perspectives spanning anthropology to sociology, cite how these universal mechanisms of misery interfere with our ability to create meaningful lives for ourselves. These travails are known as the *kleshas* ("afflictions") in yogic philosophy.

The first affliction is *avidya*, or the confusion of identifying the Self with the limitations of material existence rather than the eternally free consciousness of the Soul. Belief in the existence or idea of a "soul" may not resonate with some folks; however, it's not a prerequisite to understanding that bodies age (and youthful beauty fades), money can't buy happiness, and no one escapes tragedy or death. Still, the trappings of embodiment are so alluring that avidya feeds the other four kleshas.

Asmita refers to the further misidentification of Self and consciousness with features of "I am-ness," such as "I am this body," "I am this personality," "I am a Sagittarius." From these obfuscations of our true nature, we get further entangled in myths about ourselves and reality with the big *R*. As the web of illusion tightens around us, we seek a way out of the pressure by seeking more pleasure (*raga*) and feeling less pain (*dvesa*). Talk about opposites that attract. On their own, raga and dvesa wreak havoc in our lives, from fueling addictions to avoiding accountability for our problems. Together, they bring more misery as we struggle between holding on to what we think makes us happy and avoiding our fears. We become so saturated and sticky with grasping desire for this life, beyond the inherent biological imperative that comes with embodiment, that we get pulled further into the web. This blind greed for more and more life is known as *abhinivesa*, and it prevents us from confronting the ignorance or illusion that our consciousness somehow originates in and is bound to this earthly body.[2]

So, if not confined and defined within a body, what is the true nature of beingness? Across time, from convents to kitchen tables, folks have sought to understand this very question. Here again, yogic philosophy offers a framework in a doctrine called *pancamaya* or *pancakosha*. Explicated thousands of years ago in the Upanishads, Brahma Sutras, and Bhagavad Gita,[3] which are sacred texts of yoga, pancamaya/pancakosha foreshadows more recent discoveries and observations about homeostasis, resilience, interdependence, and consciousness. It refers to five "veils" (*maya*) or "sheaths" (*koshas*) of sentient embodiment that interact on earthly and divine planes, from the body to the eternal self. What happens in one kosha affects the others, akin to the misery-loves-company interdependence of the kleshas. The sheaths are ordered from gross to subtle, or from the directly observable to the discreet.

The first, most readily accessible layer of being is known as *anna-maya*. Composed of food, it corresponds to the tissues and structures of our physical anatomy. Body maps, postural orientation, and movement study help us discern the robustness of annamaya kosha. From this physical layer, the "anatomy" becomes less material. *Pranamaya* is the next sheath, and it is composed of the breath. The breath is classified as the essential life force, or prana, that vitalizes the material life cycle from birth to death. Since it expresses the condition of the life force, pranamaya is viewed as the energy body. *Manomaya*, composed of thought, relates to the activity of the mind—thoughts, emotions, perspectives, and beliefs. *Vijnanamaya*, composed of understanding, is the wisdom layer that expresses our heartfelt desires and truth. The deepest kosha is *anandamaya*, composed of pure joy. Known as the bliss body, it resonates most closely with the soul known as Atman.

Let's experiment with identifying each of these sheaths for ourselves right now, circumstances permitting. Set a timer for ten minutes, if you like. Adjust your body position and close your eyes, if you prefer. Close your mouth and take in an unforced, deep breath through your nose. Then sigh out the exhalation through softly parted lips. Do this twice more. Close your mouth and focus on breathing in and out through your nose without strain. If the nose breathing feels forced, part your lips slightly and try sipping the breath through an imaginary straw until you're ready to resume through your nose. Count ten rounds of inhalation and exhalation, then let go of the breath counting and check in with each of the koshas without rushing or dawdling: How does the body feel right now? How much energy does it take to breathe? Does the mind chatter match up with how I feel right now? Where do I feel my sense of self and identity in my body in this moment? Where do I sense an inner vastness right now, in this moment? After another six rounds of relaxed breath, let out an exhalation with a sigh. Open your eyes when you're ready. As you notice the residue of this brief kosha scan, consider the good news: if we are looking to alleviate our suffering as single, sentient beings or to foster peace in the world at large, we have agency. We can untangle ourselves from the knots of misery through yoga.

Patanjali outlined that the limbs of yoga provide the tools and skills to free us from the limitations of a bodily existence defined by narrow words and fear of the misunderstood. The Eight Limbs include cadenced breathing (pranayama), concentration (*dharana*), and meditation (*dhyana*) practices as well as asana. These four methods of organized awareness training energize development of the other four limbs: a stronger ethical compass (*yama*), more compassionate behavior (*niyama*), self-awareness (*pratyahara*), and integration or bliss (*samadhi*). In Patanjali's words, devoted self-study through yoga enables us to grow into our authentic oneness. He summed it up in the previously mentioned sutra, *Tada drastuh svarupe vasthanam.*[4] Whether we are seeking karmic liberation (*moksha*) or not, each of these practices yields powerful consequences across every dimension of our lives.

Yoga and Mind-Body Connection

In various fields of research, human existence is frequently described in terms of a bio-psychosocial-spiritual model of health and living, which is evocative of pancakosha doctrine. *Bio-* refers to our biology (anatomy and physiology); *psycho-*, to our emotional and mental well-being; *social,* to our relationships; and *spiritual,* to our beliefs about living and dying. Specialists in the *-ics, -ologies,* and *-sciences* measure and examine all types of biomarkers—from inflammatory factors and insulin levels in blood samples to changes in heartbeat intervals and brainwaves in sleep studies—in efforts to identify the mechanisms and triggers that affect myriad aspects of bio-psychosocial-spiritual health.

Yoga is included in a grouping of holistic health practices referred to as mind-body interventions (MBIs) or mind-body training (MBT) in clinical research. Tai chi, mindfulness-based stress reduction, progressive relaxation, and prayer fall under this umbrella as well. MBIs share several features appealing to social, health, and medical science researchers. These practices are typically low risk, cost-effective, and straightforward to adapt. At the nuts-and-bolts level, it's easy to begin a daily pranayama or restorative yoga practice with nothing more than attentive observation and breath. Furthermore, the effects of specific breathing and conscious rest techniques may be gauged in terms of objective, quantifiable changes in blood chemistry and neural activity. When combined with other data-rich metrics, such as self-reporting of symptoms, experts in fields ranging from psychology to neurology to immunology support a broadening consensus: learning to focus on breath and body sensations, as well as tuning in to the innermost dialogue of emotions, beliefs, and judgments, strengthens our connection with moment-to-moment aliveness. It is this connection that is the wellspring for resilience, wellness, and contentment.[5]

Several features of our brain-to-body, body-to-brain communication pathways make us particularly susceptible to yogic manipulation. To start, the brain comprises three extensively connected systems organized by functions and location. Planning and executive structures are located nearest the brain's surface, closer to the front and sides of the skull. These structures are collectively called the cortex. The helmetlike cortex surrounds the labeling and sorting regions of the brain, located in the deep area behind the eyes and between the ears. This inner region is home to the limbic system. Beneath the limbic system are nestled the midbrain and brain stem, which are directly connected to the spinal cord. Dubbed the reptilian brain, the primary survival systems that govern cardiovascular and respiratory function as well as autonomic nervous system activation are in the midbrain and brain stem.

The limbic system, nicknamed the emotional brain, includes structures that process and pattern emotions and bodily feelings. It includes the amygdala, which is our alert siren, and hippocampus, which is like the FAQ for threat assessment. The limbic system is connected to the cortical regions of the brain that organize and set us on courses of action. The emotional brain is simultaneously linked to the ancient autopilot regions of the midbrain and brain stem. And the trip from the emotional to the reptilian brain is shorter and faster than the trip from body to cortex.

We like to believe that the "rational" brain regions turn on first and speak the loudest, especially when circumstances go haywire. Alas, the cortex takes a backseat to its survival-prioritizing partners operating in the center and base of the brain. In addition to the neuronal connections between the limbic system and reptilian brain, we also have hormonal messengers that chemically boost or suppress the nervous system to promote feelings of safety and well-being. In other words, our brains are organized in such a way that our emotional state affects—and is affected by—our physical state of arousal or relaxation.

We are also neurologically organized for community living, courtesy of neural structures that form the social engagement system. Believe it or not, we even have a network of mirror neurons that help us mimic behavior, body language, and facial expressions so we can align ourselves with other people.[6] Curmudgeonly hermits and social butterflies alike live in the same anatomical reality: our brains—and thus, behaviors—are informed by the folks around us. This tend-and-befriend system helps monitor how safe we feel and the degree to which we trust our companions.

The social engagement system, in the midbrain structure called the medulla oblongata, is linked to the limbic system and brain stem. A pair of vagus nerves, which is one of a dozen cranial nerve pairs, emerges from this region. Cranial nerves are wired to the organs of perception and sensation—eyes, ears, skin, and so on—as well as the muscles affecting facial expression, speech, chewing, and swallowing. The vagus nerves are the longest of these and detect sensory input in just about every organ system, casting a wide net from brain stem to belly. Some 80 percent of their fibers are sensory, body-to-brain pathways. The other fibers are motor bundles from brain to body, helping move the face, mouth, and throat; and parasympathetic, relating to the rate of cardiovascular and respiratory activity.

The vagus nerves gather intel from consciously and subconsciously perceived stimuli, gut feelings (such as heartbreak, clenched stomach); tone of voice (a soothing lullaby, an ominous growl, and so on); and nonverbal cues like facial expressions and posture (for instance, a friendly smile with an open and relaxed body position, an intimidating scowl with crossed arms and a turned shoulder). They also function as the switchboard operators for autonomic nervous system regulation. Based on safety perception, the vagus nerves either apply the brakes of parasympathetic rest-digest-repair-reproduce processes or allow a cascade of sympathetic arousal responses to rev up.

In sum, when the social engagement system indicates that we are in sync with the goings-on around us, we feel alert yet relaxed. However, if we feel threatened, various physiological processes lead to increased tension and vigilance. Thus, we're prepared to escape, hide, or defend ourselves if social engagement responses such as pacifying displays of cooperation fail to keep the peace. In a worst-case scenario, we are unable to move away from or otherwise nullify danger. We have no choice but to endure, so the vagus nerves slam on the parasympathetic brakes and bring us to a complete stop. We become immobilized and "play dead." If we're lucky, the threat ends and we return to our embodied awareness, harmed but alive. Sometimes, in fact, the immobilization response is so complete that it leads to actual death.[7]

Luckily, an expanding catalog of quantitative and qualitative research confirms the friendly utility of yoga practice to improve body-to-brain, brain-to-body functioning. Pranayama, concentration, and meditation techniques correlate with important gains in emotional self-regulation, executive and cognitive functioning, and overall stress resilience. Research pertaining to the physiological effects of pranayama demonstrates reduced blood levels of biomarkers specific to sustained or chronic sympathetic nervous system arousal at different intervals postpractice. As mentioned previously, there's significant data indicating that asana helps individuals mediate chronic pain and impediments to movement akin to other forms of physical exercise. Studies about restorative yoga indicate its efficacy as a strategy to reduce symptoms of anxiety as well as fatigue, exhaustion, and burnout. The impacts of daily meditation practice are also well documented. A dedicated period of structured quietude supports positive changes across the board, from how well we remember the actions of Plank Pose to how fluent we feel in expressing our emotions, needs, and wants.[8]

A spider-limbed yoga practice builds bidirectional connections between body and brain. Data indicate that asana, pranayama, and meditative training leverages neuroplasticity throughout the brain and neural pathways affecting movement and sensory awareness as well as perception of well-being.[9] Furthermore, studies show we don't have to spend hours each day holding Plank Pose or counting breaths to feel safe and centered. Each of us knows how ten rounds of breath can help us find our terra firma and restore a sense of agency. By dedicating only five minutes per day to pranayama and twenty minutes to restorative yoga, we add time-efficient brain builders that fill out our self-care repertoire with functional gifts that keep on giving on and off the mat.

Regulate and Rewire

The equipment for meditative practice is modest. The essential condition is to find a place that feels safe; when you are there, you feel confident that you can sit or lie down quietly. If conditions allow, you might close your eyes or cover them with a light cloth or eye bag. A timer of some sort is useful, though counting a strand of prayer beads or rounds of breath also serves as a tracker. It's important to explicitly schedule pranayama and other contemplative practices into your daily routine. Personally, I start and end each day with ten minutes of pranayama and seated focusing techniques. I also have a thirty-minute block in my midday schedule for restoratives, which I piggyback onto a meal or snack.

No matter what, practice needs to be . . . well, practical. For most of us, practicality necessitates prioritization—and a dose of inventiveness. You have time for asana, pranayama, concentration, and meditation practice as long as you designate it as part of your day.

For example, take the same walk every day? During the first five minutes or time it takes to reach a landmark, focus your attention on the sensations of body and breath as you walk. Have a cup of tea or coffee every day at the same time? Practice three minutes of conscious breathing or a different pranayama technique while waiting for it to steep or brew. Do you press the snooze button when your alarm wakes you? Use the snooze interval for meditative engagement—with breath, body, energy level, and so on. Heck, you can even do many of the core stabilization exercises in bed, so you could use that snooze time for some body learning. In other words, how we use time reflects what we value. Put self-connection at the top of the value list and plug it in to your daily routine.

More intentionality may be necessary to break the code on adding a demarcated period of restorative yoga. While you certainly do not need to build an elaborate napping nest, you will feel more comfortable if you are able to take the time to support yourself with blankets, pillows or bolsters, and blocks. Consider feeding two birds with one seed by adding a twenty-minute cushion to your bedtime routine to establish a restorative habit. After all, we must sleep at some point, and restorative yoga has positive effects on how quickly we fall asleep and the duration of sleep. During this presleep time, you get settled in bed, set a timer for twenty minutes, and meander through a body scan. All the while, the nervous system is slowing down toward sleep.

A hurdle frequently encountered during meditative practice is positional and bodily discomfort, just like in active asana. And just like in active asana, we heed the body's messages about feeling cold or warm; numb hands and feet; tense shoulders and jaws; and especially pain in the neck, low back, hips, and knees. Uncomfortable sensation is the body requesting help. Remember how the nervous system responds when help is unavailable or denied? The stress pathways get activated and stay that way until a felt sense of safety is restored.

When we take actions that reduce the disruption of pain, we rewire the nervous system to recognize how to feel relief. Several studies show that an emphasis on propping the body to feel steady, relaxed, and still for restorative yoga practice changes physiologic reactivity to pain and its attached emotional disturbances.[10] By learning to cushion our bodies, we unclog the pathways to other feelings and sensations active in the present moment. With consistent practice, the limbic and social engagement systems move into sync, and we feel enjoyable shifts in body and spirit.

The following three practices are meant to seduce you into stillness. They build on common sleep positions, so they're familiar as well as bed-friendly. Seriously, if the only time you can find for quiet is in bed at the start or end of your day, do these practices in bed. Combine the pranayama technique with the restorative yoga poses. The added perk is an opportunity to experiment with ways to improve sleep comfort. Pillows and blankets can become bolsters and substitute for blocks to add height. Bath towels can fill in for blankets. Ideally you have enough props to support your head, neck and shoulders, wrists and hands, legs, ankles, and feet. Think of Goldilocks again and gather the props that will help you create a just-right nest for yourself.

● ● ●

Supported Side-Lying Corpse Pose (Savasana)

PROPS: Nonskid mat, 5 blankets, 2 bolsters or large pillows, a lightweight eye cover, a timer

All paths lead to Corpse Pose, on and off the mat. Abhinivesa daily reminds us of the irrevocable fact of mortality—and most of us don't like thinking about it. Corpse Pose trains us to accept the ultimate stillness by holding the space to notice and identify the constant flow of what is active in us, from the pleasant to the unpleasant, the glaringly obvious to the persistently evasive. As we become more attuned to ourselves, we come to recognize and understand that absolutely everything is ever changing and impermanent. Given how fervently we cling to beliefs of certitude about the nature of how things are, this disidentification process takes a lot of time and practice. Thankfully we can do it lying down.

Side-Lying Corpse Pose is practiced while resting on the preferred side of your body. Place a bifold or fourfold blanket on top of your sticky mat for added cushioning and insulation. Make a fourfold blanket by folding a blanket in half widthwise, then lengthwise. Next, take a second blanket and turn it into an eightfold: fold it in half widthwise, then lengthwise, then widthwise and lengthwise again. The result will be a blanket with eight layers. Repeat this folding process with another blanket. This pair of eightfold blankets will become the support for your head, neck, and shoulders, so place them at the head of the mat.

Next, if you do not have 2 bolsters or large pillows, prepare a fourfold blanket and roll it into a thick log. This will become a bolster to hug. You may also want to make a second blanket log to place against the back of your body. Next, prepare another fourfold blanket and fold it to fit between your legs from knee to foot. Save the last blanket as a body cover. Have a small, lightweight cloth nearby.

With the eightfold blankets at the head of the mat and the bolsters along the sides of the mat, sit in the middle and ease yourself onto the preferred side of your body. Adjust your pelvis so you are resting in front of the greater trochanter rather than rolling backward or pressing on it directly. Bend your hips and knees comfortably, and place the folded blanket between your lower legs from knee to ankle. You may need to add another folded blanket. Remember to adjust the props based on your body's signals for space and/or support.

Adjust your lower shoulder by reaching toward the wall in front of you, so you rest on the armpit-edge of the shoulder blade rather than the upper arm bone. Pull the body-covering blanket up to your waist or hips. Reach behind and pull the bolster, pillow, or rolled blanket against your back. Then turn your attention to the head support. The eightfold blankets need to fill the space between the mat and your head and neck, without forcing your head to tilt or allowing it to droop. Your chin needs to be gently cradled at the top of your throat without affecting the swallow or breath.

Angle the stacked eightfold blankets to mirror the angle of your chin. Next, adjust the layers of the head blankets to fill in around the contours of your head and neck and the top of your shoulders. Don't shove the blankets to make space. Simply press and tuck the blanket folds until you feel the weight of your head, neck, and shoulders cradled in the blanket nest.

Next, pull the "hugging" bolster into the front of your body and rest your arms as you prefer. To increase arm comfort, place a small, folded towel under the wrist and hand of your bottom arm. Lifting the hand in this way often creates ease all the way up to the neck and jaw. Also, place a small, rolled towel between your upper arm and side ribs, near the armpit. The rolled towel helps the head of the arm bone sit more comfortably in the shoulder socket. Pull the covering blanket up so you're covered from your shoulders to your feet. Start a timer for 15 to 20 minutes, cover your eyes with a lightweight cloth, and readjust as necessary. Allow yourself to settle and shift to nose breathing. Count 10 relaxed rounds of breath and then adjust your props and position if you need more comfort. Resettle and resume breathing in and out through your nose without strain.

Until the timer goes off, lie still and focus your attention on the sensations of the breath. Feel your body breathing itself. Notice how and where your skin stretches with inhalation and slackens with exhalation. Notice the brief pauses, the little deaths, at the top of each inhalation and bottom of each exhalation. When concentration on the breath fades, note the break in focus and redirect your attention to the breath sounds and movements. Listen as well to the words that skitter into your field of attention. These words may correspond to changes in breath sounds, sensations, or emotions, so pay particular attention to where words live in or stimulate your body.

When the timer goes off, allow your senses to gently open to the space around you. Ease yourself up slowly to a comfortable seated position when ready. Take a few rounds of breath before moving on. As mentioned elsewhere in this guide, you may find it helpful to keep a meditation or practice journal to reflect on the discoveries revealed in the deep world of Corpse Pose.

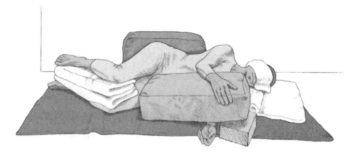

FIGURE 7.1. Supported Side-Lying Corpse Pose

* * *

Even Breathing (Sama Vritti) in Supported Supine Pranayama Position

PROPS: Nonskid mat, 5 blankets, 1 large towel, a lightweight eye cover, a timer

One of the most centering, harmony-restoring things we can do for ourselves is practice slow, controlled pranayama. When we focus on the sensations and movements of breath, we are unable to divert our attention from how we feel here and now. The breath is a powerful magnet that holds us together in the present. It's a surefire reality check. Pranayama is also one of the most portable yoga techniques in that it can be done anywhere, anytime, with nothing but the willingness and capacity to affix our attention to the breath. However, so we develop the concentration skills for pranayama, we will practice in a supine position specifically designed to reduce bodily, emotional, and mental tension that inhibits breath. Pranayama involves exploration of the phases, ratios, and pace of inhalation, exhalation, and retention. As we grow in practice, we experiment more freely with patterned rhythms. For now, we will study Even Breathing, which involves inhaling and exhaling at the same rate. Retaining the automatic pause between inhalation and exhalation at the same rate may be added after twelve weeks of daily practice. More on that later. Begin with a rate of 5-count inhalation/5-count exhalation.

Set up the mat with a fourfold blanket as before. Next, prepare the back-body supports that will gently lift your rib cage by supporting your body from the top of your sacrum past the crown of your head. Take a fourfold blanket and fold it in thirds lengthwise. Place this blanket lengthwise on the center of the mat. Prepare another blanket the same way and place it on top of its twin. Situate the top blanket so that the bottom blanket's tail end is exposed. The lumbopelvic ends of the blankets form a slope to meet the natural curve of the body. Fold the head end of the top blanket onto itself to help cushion and support your head and neck.

Place a thick blanket roll near the knee space of the mat. A bolster works as well, as long as it isn't so thick as to crowd your hips, pelvic floor, and deep belly. Roll a large towel into a slim log to support the Achilles notches at the back of your ankles. Have a lightweight eye cover and body blanket nearby.

Sit in the center of the mat with the tail end of the bottom blanket filling the curve where your sacrum and buttocks turn under. Place the thick blanket roll or bolster behind your knees and the rolled towel behind your ankles. Pull the body-covering blanket up to your waist. Then plant your hands by your hips, draw your belly button in and up, and roll your body down onto the long blanket supports.

Fiddle with the top blanket flap to fill in the space around your neck and to lift the crown of your head gently until your chin is lower than your forehead. Once your head feels steady and comfortable, cover your eyes, and pull the blanket up to cover your shoulders and arms. With an inhalation, move your arms away from your body without shrugging your shoulders or turning your arm bones in or out. Remember, place folded towels or blankets under your wrists and hands for added support.

Start a timer set for 7 minutes. Allow yourself to settle and shift to nose breathing. Count 10 relaxed rounds of breath. After an exhalation, inhale for a count of 5—not too fast, not too slow. Slide through the phase-switching pause and exhale for the same count of 5. Again, don't linger in retention. Continue to inhale for 5, exhale for 5 until the timer goes off. If you lose track, reconnect to inhaling and exhaling smoothly and evenly for a count of 5. When you hear the timer, finish the round of breath you are engaged with and then inhale slowly. Relax through the exhalation. Allow the breath to establish its own rhythm, and when you're ready, roll to the side that's most comfortable for you. Rest for as long as you like, then slowly sit up. Take a few rounds of breath before moving on. As your pranayama skill grows, consider extending the length of practice up to 30 minutes on days when you have more schedule latitude.

Later, as your body allows, experiment with a different pattern, starting with a 7-minute practice. After three months of relaxed, nose-only 5:5 Even Breathing, switch to a 5-count inhalation/5-count retention/5-count exhalation. Pay exquisite attention to your heart rhythm and rate in this new pattern, especially during the 5-count holds. If you feel your heart racing, skipping, or clustering beats, let go of the retention. If you feel a rush into or out of inhalation or exhalation following retention, take 2 rounds of natural breath through the nose between each round of 5:5:5. If the strain persists, reduce the pause duration until it is eased. The key to pranayama is that it resonates with the nervous system rather than agitates it. Strain or force in the breath during practice is a sign that the nervous system needs a gentler approach.

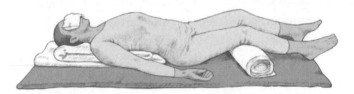

FIGURE 7.2. Supported Supine Pranayama Position

● ● ●

Stonehenge Restorative

PROPS: Nonskid mat, 3 blankets, 2 blocks, 1 bolster or
2 large pillows, a lightweight eye cover, a timer

The third contemplative practice is restorative yoga. It's a receptive method of prop-supported asana that promotes deep physical and mental relaxation. The more time you give this practice, the more benefits you'll accumulate in higher levels of bonding hormones such as oxytocin and neurotransmitters like serotonin. At a minimum, give restorative practice 20 minutes to allow the vagal brakes to engage and the autonomic nervous system to move into parasympathetic eminence (an alert yet relaxed state). Since many folks experience low back pain at some point in their lives, the pose affectionately termed "Stonehenge" offers welcome relief. It's a relatively simple setup, too.

Place a fourfold blanket on top of the mat for padding and warmth. Next, take a second blanket and turn it into an eightfold. Place it at the top end of the mat to serve as a head, neck, and shoulder support.

Take two blocks and place them upright like pillars, about sitting bone–width apart, at the tail end of the fourfold blanket. Place a bolster with its wide, flat side across the tops of the blocks. See the resemblance to those well-known rock structures? Finally, fold a blanket in half widthwise once and again, so you have a wide fourfold. Place another blanket to cover your body and a lightweight eye cover nearby.

Sit in the center of the mat and place your legs on top of the bolster. Adjust the flesh of your calf muscles as needed by pulling them outward. Ease your upper body down onto the mat and roll your thigh bones gently inward to seat the heads of the thigh bones in the hip sockets. Next, take the wide fourfold blanket and lay it over your pelvis from the rim to the pubic bones. Roll a little to one side and tuck a bit of the blanket under the lifted hip, then do the same under the other hip. Tuck the blanket snugly around your pelvis, across the greater trochanters, like a swaddle. Readjust as needed.

Customize the head support next. Slide the eightfold blanket under your head and neck to the tops of your shoulders and tuck the blanket layers into the curves. Fold the top corners of the blanket under to gently lift the top of your head and lower your chin. Set a timer for 20 to 30 minutes. Pull a blanket over your body, cover your eyes, and pull your arms under the blanket. Place your arms far enough from your body to allow the side ribs to move with the breath.

Direct your attention to the body breathing itself. Notice the skin sensations that accompany inhalation and exhalation. Notice the brief pauses between breath phases. Notice the beating of your heart, the sound of your beating heart.

Now, scan every region of your body, part by part, guided by the body maps we have drafted for ourselves. Move the attention deliberately through each part, nook, cranny, and region. Resist the temptation to loiter. Then sense your body front and back, side to side, upper half and lower half, and as a whole.

Abide in the awareness of your body until the timer chimes. Then open your senses to the space around you. Stretch gently through your arms and legs, if desired. Roll to the side that is most comfortable for you, breathing into the skin of your back. Ease yourself up slowly to a comfortable seated position when you're ready. Take a few rounds of breath before moving on.

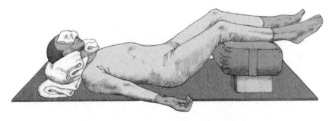

FIGURE 7.3. Stonehenge Restorative

Plugged In and (Em)Powered Up

Every move, breath, thought, and belief is influenced in varying degrees, conscious and otherwise, by our emotional state. We grow in confidence the more often we invite the residues and sources of feelings and sensations into awareness. Meditative inquiries lead us to routes in our bodies that reveal and heal wounds of the heart, soma, and psyche as well as liberate energy and spirit. The cumulative effects of practice start leaking out into life off the mat. Unless you want to, you will not become a hemp sandal–wearing vegan because of yoga practice. You will, however, become a more attuned, sensitive person to some degree or another.

8

Yoga Forward

GO YOUR OWN WAY

Remember when life's path is steep
to keep your mind even.
—Horace[1]

Yoga practice leads to more connectivity in the body-to-brain, brain-to-body networks anatomically, functionally, and intuitively—sandals or no. The body and brain wire together more intimately and extensively, the threads of sensations and feelings weaving a growing neural web of awareness and cohesion. Through steady practice, we activate more and different regions of the brain, improving sensory perception, processing, and patterning. We develop stability, strength, and controlled range of motion. We feel, recognize, and become conversant in a broadening spectrum of our psychosomatic reality. We become more sensitive while simultaneously less reactive.

Sometimes we become so synced up that we feel liberated from the boundaries of physical existence. These episodes represent early stages in a process of awareness expansion called *samadhi* in the Yoga Sutras. The more often we practice, the sooner we feel these flashes of transcendence. Ironically, we usually describe this sense of boundlessness in terms of the infinitesimal.

Think of a time in your life when you resonated with the knowledge that your individual life is akin to a single grain of sand, bit of stardust, or drop in the sea. Remember how peaceful and perfect those moments felt? These interludes of atomic consciousness reveal the discrepancies between identifying with fleeting, albeit tenacious beliefs about who/what/why we are based on the constant hum of busyness and opening our attention to the aliveness beyond words, breath, and bone. Recognizing the vastness within and beyond us, through asana, pranayama, and restoratives, nourishes our "trust-in-the-gut" mechanism. Feeling the universal vibe confirms what we know but have forgotten: Everything Is Perfect. We remember that perfection when we attune to and trust our embodied feelings. The more we practice, the more we remember and the easier it becomes to trust ourselves. The cup of contentment runneth over when filled from that wellspring of inner peace.

We can visit a place of peace and harmony within ourselves directly on a daily basis. The lessons shared in this book are designed for finding the center of groundedness within every one of us. All that's necessary is practice. Again, simple but not easy.

Choices, Choices, Choices

One of my early teachers, Nancy Ford-Kohne, often stated, "Yoga is the conscious choice of the difficult." Over the years I have interpreted that assertion in several ways, frequently to castigate myself into a punishing pattern of overwork and underappreciation. Thankfully, my arms got tired of holding up the weight of all that externally driven yet self-imposed judgment. And my brain changed. It grew bigger in the sense that I have an increased capacity and a higher tolerance to hold more of myself at once.

Yoga practice trains us to choose presence consciously, to feel fully embodied in the present moment, right now, over and over again. To be present feels difficult when we blame and shame ourselves for not living up to someone else's definition of success or acceptability. Presence feels difficult when we become discouraged and broken down by thoughts about the constant vigilance and monotony that seem part and parcel of showing up all the time. Choosing to stay synced in body, breath, and mind also feels difficult when the present moment is judged to be too much. The assessment of feeling overwhelmed or threatened may be an accurate reflection of current circumstances or an evocation of past pain and its coping mechanisms.

Regardless of the source, we can resolve all types of difficulties—from the mundane to the existential—by locating, labeling, and feeling the sensations, emotions, thoughts, and beliefs that attend them. We practice watching them shift at their own pace, without force or strain, just like the rise and fall of the breath. This is how we eventually let go of attachments to the ephemera of our body-bound business and tap into the lifeblood of universal wholeness, that incomprehensible yet palpable presence of everything and nothing. We learn to observe the inherent, organic constancy of change within ourselves.

Once we have faith in the reliability of impermanence, we expand our capacity and curiosity for the harmony that comes from unwinding and feel our flow in this chiasmatic confluence of the gross to subtle, individual to cosmic. Make no mistake, we still need to practice every day. We know by now that every Plank Pose is new each time it's practiced. However, the growing reliability of our presence in the here and now fosters ease in our undertakings. We still need to work to maintain connectivity between all our layers, but the work itself is more efficient and readily yields gems of insight and mystery that often lead to pathways of peace and gratitude.

An Attitude of Gratitude

We simply cannot struggle through obstacles and restrictions, whatever their nature. Struggle comes from an imposed sense of urgency. Running around while flapping our gums and wobbling our heads delays or even prevents recovery and reparation. To make it through the wilderness of this life's journey in one piece, we need to stop, observe our surroundings, assess our condition, and then plan. In other words, slow down, stabilize, and then move. Just like we need core stabilization to ensure motion control, we need attitude adjustment to ensure a healthy mindset. This entails a commitment to practicing every single day to become stable in habit and observance. We also need to give ourselves permission to do what we feel up to, when we feel up to doing it. This is not a pass to do the bare minimum. It's an invitation to rely on your practice to become aware of and responsive to your own rhythms.

Yoga philosophy provides perspective on how to nurture a commitment to practice, which is a necessary condition for reaping its rewards. Two niyama serve as powerful foci that converge into an attitude of gratitude: *tapas* and *svadhyaya*. Both act as a specific practice and process of personal discipline.

Tapas is a burning zeal for disentangling from illusion and a process of eliminating that which no longer serves us in our quest for inner and outer harmony. It's the get-up-and-go, the impetus and motivation to step onto the mat and stay there, if only for a minute. Tapas is built by doing, meaning to feel zeal you must zealously do the things that perpetuate it. In a nutshell, you gotta give to get. You also need to know what you are giving and getting, hence svadhyaya.

Svadhyaya refers to self-inquiry, the study of yourself to understand yourself. It is the practice of tracking the currents of our emotions, thoughts, and beliefs by way of asana, pranayama, and restoratives. Since the mind runs a turbulent gamut, we benefit from learning more about how to contextualize the products of our thinking and feeling brains. Thus, svadhyaya also refers to the study of sacred texts. Let's face it, sometimes we all need outside guidance to cut through the static.

While this book is centered around the idea of the body as guide, given its role as an entity, conduit, and crossroad of existence, other sources may inform our self-inquiry and offer respite in times of doubt, fatigue, and instability. If you have not done so already, purchase or borrow a copy of *The Yoga Sutras of Patanjali*. There are a bunch of translations, so peruse a few and choose one that speaks to your gut.

Maybe you are more inclined toward contemporary voices about self-knowing and self-connection. Authors from Brené Brown to Pema Chödrön have provided a plethora of insightful, engaging books to support self-inquiry. What is important about this aspect of svadhyaya is that you connect to inspiration. Consider studying archetypes that reflect qualities of character and presence you want to emulate—or even avoid. A cautionary tale every now and then tends to reinvigorate our attention. Stories about scary manifestations remind us of the coexistence of lesser traits and moral pitfalls. They support accountability without making it personal or ad hominem.

Most important of all, have fun. Turn that frown upside down. Play on the mat. Try the variations for each exercise. Make up some of your own, guided by the information in the early chapters about bones and balance. Breathe. Laugh. Listen to music. Turn on a fan or heater. Savor the sensations and shifts of body and breath. Practice outside, inside, in the dark, on a rooftop. Soak your heart in gratitude for the opportunity to simply feel alive.

Independent but Not Alone

Being human entails being in relationship all the time, even when we're convinced we are alone. In its simplest distillation, *yoga* is a verb that describes the collective actions of being. The word *yug* means "to yoke, to bind together." The practices of yoga's Eightfold Path bind the layers of our being in relationship to the layers of self and to one another—from family to polity to life, death, and every-thing in between.

Calibrating interactions, internally and externally, entails reflec-tion after action. This is another way of saying that slowing down and checking in keeps us rolling down the road. We miss so much information, intuition, and experience in our hurry to get ahead. Ambition really does blind us. It's a form of toxic motivation that runs us down and washes us out. I don't know where or what we are rushing toward, given that no matter where we go, there we are. We might as well make our own way intentionally, taking in the scenery as we go. I learned that lesson repeatedly from my older students, especially thanks to a pair of then-septuagenarians many years ago.

I used to see these ladies weekly, just the two of them, in my home studio. Our sessions were a minimum of ninety minutes and sometimes two hours. They'd been neighbors and friends of fifty years or so by the time I came into the picture. Both were avid gardeners, book club members, and feminists. We used to go out to supper and live theater performances together, beyond the mat. These friends were also opposites, and sometimes they would clash. Then they would return to peace in their own language. It was so heartwarming to be with them.

One was born and had spent most of her life in the mid-Atlantic region, primarily in the suburbs of Washington, D.C. She raised three children as a single parent when that was a family configura-tion even less accepted than it is today. The other was a child-free widow. She had emigrated from the Philippines to the United States in early midlife with her American husband. She had survived the horrors of the Japanese occupation during World War II. She taught me that we carry freedom within our bodies, and no government or organization has the power to either confer or deprive the rights of liberty even when they have their boots on our backs.

We worked together on the mat for several years. When the ladies began with me, they professed an interest in improving their balance, reducing fall risk, building core stability, and doing some strength work. We laid out some grand plans together. I was so enthusiastic about helping them with their achy parts and issues. I had all these certifications to work with scoliosis and osteoporosis and so on. I had been teaching for ten years at that point. And soon I was schooled in the best possible way when it came to giving myself and other folks time on the mat to link up attention with sensation, feeling with emotion, belief with thought, and action with intention.

My habit is to solve things, to work the problems. If I am not doing something, I am somehow failing in ethics and effort. (Ahem, patriarchal capitalism, thanks for the jacked-up nervous system and skew toward self-punishment.) As a result, I have gained some notoriety among students who know me: I tend to be something of a firehose when it comes to spraying information. I also have been known to truncate or entirely skip Corpse Pose after teaching anything other than restoratives and pranayama explicitly. Mind you, I am a certified restorative and iRest Level 1 teacher. All my science and experiential background aside, I am a Corpse Pose thief.

Fortunately, these wise women made it clear to me that I could and would not get away with skipping this pose when it came to our time together. Not only would every session include Corpse Pose or another type of restorative, that rest period was going to be at least thirty minutes long. I quickly came to delight in tucking them in as well as teaching them to adjust their props and positioning for comfort during rest and sleep. As we folded blankets, both would softly share stories of their fatigue and concerns or troubles with me. Then they would show me how to restore themselves by closing their eyes and settling into their breath. Those ladies napped with reckless abandon, like my children, who were still small at the time.

From asana to pranayama, my duo of vibrant, tired, courageous women gently countered my tendencies toward overexertion and showed me to tune in to the wisdom of my own body. The histories they shared with me—some horrific in brutality and inhumanity—mustered the recognition for me that life is an ultramarathon and running it like a sprint is a common folly. Why was I in such a hurry? And why were these old ladies, who had more time behind them than ahead, so content to simply go along at their own inclination?

Their lack of "work" and sheer enjoyment of moving—and not moving—was stunning to me. There were all these rules, which I knew so well and shared so openly. This pair of compatriots ignored them. They simply kept their attention on the breath and let it move them. Or they laid down. There was a potent dignity in their leisureliness. As they became more still, more of their aliveness became available to their awareness.

Their brilliant and vexing nonconformity was as revelatory as it was karmic. They taught me that I did not have to entertain my students with doing. My role in class was much simpler and far more satisfying. I saw that I needed to teach fewer rules about asana aesthetics—how to do a pose—and invite more somatosensory autonomy. That meant I needed to see the forest and the trees, so I could help folks cocreate the conditions for asana to emerge of its own accord. And that meant I had to slow down—way, way down—on my mat and in class. It meant becoming not only comfortable but also passionately curious about independence and allyship.

Each of us is our own person. We make our way as best we can, even when it seems the world is falling apart. Trust your gut and team up with others who are growing into their guts as well. This doesn't mean we have to be best friends forever. It simply means we are all poor, wayfaring strangers, and we create joy and safety when we inquire about and respect one another's needs and wants. We are all running around in the woods, trying to make it to Grandma's house, and the paths of fellow soul seekers will cross. When they do, walk together for a while. Break out the trail mix and water, help tend to any wounds, and share your stories. We don't have to agree about anything. All that's necessary is to accept that each of us will eventually go our own way, independent but not alone for long.

Aim for the North Star

Anatomy and kinesiology study helped me learn to decode the structural clues and root movements that influence how each of us expresses asana. The deciphering seems daunting at first, but stick with it. The purpose of the body- and grid-mapping activities is not to know or predict all potential body shapes and movement patterns. We practice landmark sighting and postural interpretation to see clues and tendencies, to illuminate factors that determine—to one degree or another—how we unleash the sacred forms of asana from the center of our bodies and beings. Repetitive exposure to different folks will keep you engaged for years. Bodies are never boring!

Once we get a sense of how we are shaped and pulled around by gravity, it feels intrinsically reasonable that we need to get organized in our bellies. Certainly, we recognize the center mass of the body as tissues, organs, and bones. Now we understand that this center is more than physical mass. It's our North Star.

The pelvis is the source of our locomotion and progress. By developing dynamic stability around the anatomical basin of the body, we build the power and control to swing ourselves around with more tolerance for load and error. We stop wasting energy trying to move ourselves from the actions of smaller parts better suited to other, often more subtle tasks. We find our track and stay on it.

Dedicated rest periods and several minutes of breath awareness practice put all the trail blazing and moving around in context: these interludes of peace and quiet help us rebound, reimagine our state of affairs, and repair wear and tear. Each of us has a body where we live, no matter how much or little we feel it. *Teach People, Not Poses* is offered as a "big tent event" for stepping onto the mat on your own terms, in the context of your unique anatomy and experience. It's an exhortation to engage in asana, pranayama, and contemplative rest every single day as an act of devotion that celebrates living in your own gravitational and psychic center. May the lessons shared meet you where you are and carry you along to wherever you hope to be. Namaste.

ACKNOWLEDGMENTS

I owe many debts of gratitude. This book took me two years to write. Yoga evangelist and science nerd that I am, I had so much in my head to sort out. I rewrote the manuscript multiple times—and laid out three more books in the process. My nearest and dearest heard all about every single draft. Some read early manuscripts, others listened and talked through my ideas, often while I was sporting earbuds and tromping around in the woods with my trustworthy hound. Several did some heavy lifting, to see me through periods of dismay, imposter syndrome, and writer's block. I thank you and love you all. In alphabetical order because I like tidy lists: Angela, Be, Carol, Debra, Ellen, Heather, Judith, Lizzie, Kristen, Meg, Nicole, and Shawn.

I extend my love and gratitude to all the yoga-curious and yoga-committed people who joined me through the height of the COVID-19 pandemic for monthly online *Asana Labs*. Folks from Australia to Taiwan and across the United States gathered with me, and my digital host Lili, in "the lab." I refined the core training series based on the observations and data I gathered from the sessions and follow-up conversations. I also got to torment my husband of thirty years on the mat, on camera, and that was more fun for me than I should admit. All the years of trying to entice Reuben onto the mat and it turns out all he needed was an audience.

Lili, by the way, also illustrated this book! You rock, Lili, and I appreciate your decades of graphic design, print, and yoga experience.

Your patience, especially when it came to my nitpicky attention to detail, was a true gift to me, the hyper nerd. Thank you for all the hours on Zoom as we meticulously refined the avatars. I am still convinced that you are some sort of art witch—and I dig your magic!

My gratitude goes to my editor at Shambhala, Beth Frankl. It has been a dream of mine since age thirteen (!) to write a book and you helped me realize it. I have learned so much from you, and you helped me in ways I never expected when it came to writing. Your heart-centered communication, professionalism, and willingness to facilitate my creativity while keeping me on track has been rewarding beyond measure. I can't believe this is my book. Thank you, thank you, thank you!

Special thanks also to my fellow PTA parent, Laura Marshall, for taking my headshots. You know how much I hate to have my picture taken. You made it enjoyable, and it was delightful to reminisce about our parenting foibles as we wandered around Huntley Meadow Park. I also call out again to my dear friend Angela Russell of Salon deZen in Alexandria, Virginia. Not only has she listened to me for years on and off the mat but Angela also got me photo ready. Were it not for her ministrations, I would have looked like something the cat dragged in.

Speaking of cats, Penelope, my orange tabby, is a dedicated keyboard disrupter and monitor obscurer. She is a coffee thief and dog tormentor. I have long maintained that Penelope represents my suppressed antisocial willfulness. How I adore that she shines this mirror for me! Since she takes care of agitation, I can focus on pacification and unification. Her insistent narcissism offered me opportunities to prioritize life happening now and give it some kind pats and kisses.

Kira, my gorgeous Dobe/greyhound rescue hound, also helped me write this book. She was with me on every walk as I thought through conundrums and word-smithed in my brain. She slept in my office during late nights and got up with me for early mornings. She reminded me to take love breaks and connect to my inner refuge when she decided I had been staring at a screen for too long.

Not only does Kira help me feel safe but she also reminds to play and be silly. We spent countless hours at the dog park, refilling my laugh tank. My college-age children like to say that Kira is my favorite child. They're not wrong.

Last and most importantly, I share my love, gratitude, and relief with my family. My brother, parents, auntie, cousins, and in-laws have been ceaseless in their support and enthusiasm for this book. In fact, my dad is the person who gave me a copy of the Bhagavad Gita when I was fourteen years old. Each of you has cared for me in your own way. I love you for it.

To Jacob and Emma, you are my heart walking around on the planet. Kira may be my favorite, but y'all are the jam in my jelly roll. I am so proud of the young adults you have become. I step onto my mat every day to be more present and responsive to you. Thank you for helping me become a better bucket.

To Reuben, I love you. You have listened with varying degrees of interest to my near-incessant chatter about yoga, anatomy, kinesiology, health, and wellness for decades. Throw in the politics and activism, trauma and healing, adventures and travels, shortcomings and strengths, and we have been on a wild ride. I know we like to joke about me being high maintenance, high reward. But I also know you love me in all my weirdness and intensity. You have made it abundantly clear that you like me, too. You have done this when I have not liked, much less loved myself. Through it all, we have stuck together and built a blessed life with our peeps. Thank you for being my person. This one is for you.

NOTES

Chapter 1. Yoga Curious: Where Practice Begins

1. Lovelle Drachman, "Quotable Quote," *goodreads*, n.d., https://www
.goodreads.com/quotes/8753925-blessed-are-the-curious-for-they-shall
-have-adventures.

Chapter 2. Lay of the Land: Body Landmarks for Asana

1. J. R. R. Tolkien, *The Lord of the Rings: The Fellowship of the Ring* (New
York: Del Rey Mass Market Edition, 2012), 82.

Chapter 3. Shaped by Gravity: Anatomy, Movement, and Posture

1. Albert Einstein, "Albert Einstein Quotes," *BrainyQuotes*, 2022, www
.brainyquote.com/quotes/albert_einstein_106912.

Chapter 4. Body in Motion: The Pelvis Points North

1. Cheryl Strayed, *Brave Enough* (New York: Alfred A. Knopf, 2015), 4.
2. Diane Lee and Linda-Joy Lee, "The Functional Lumbopelvic-Hip Complex," chap. 4 in *The Pelvic Girdle: An Integration of Clinical Expertise
and Research*, 4th ed. (Edinburgh and New York: Elsevier/Churchill
Livingstone, 2011).
3. For more in-depth study of the anatomical sling systems of the body,
refer to Thomas W. Myers, *Anatomy Trains: Myofascial Meridians for
Manual Therapists and Movement Professionals*, 4th ed. (Edinburgh:
Elsevier, 2020).
4. Sabrina Youkhana, Catherine M. Dean, Moa Wolff, Catherine Sher-
rington, and Anne Tiedemann, "Yoga-Based Exercise Improves Balance

and Mobility in People Aged 60 and Over: A Systematic Review and Meta-analysis," *Age and Ageing* 45, no. 1 (January 2016): 21–29, https://doi.org/10.1093/ageing/afv175.

5. Bianca P. Acevedo, Sarah Pospos, and Helen Lavretsky, "The Neural Mechanisms of Meditative Practices: Novel Approaches for Healthy Aging," *Current Behavioral Neuroscience Reports* 3, no. 4 (2016): 328–39, www.ncbi.nlm.nih.gov/pmc/articles/PMC5110576/; Michaela C. Pascoe, David R. Thompson, and Chantal F. Ski, "Yoga, Mindfulness-Based Stress Reduction and Stress-Related Physiological Measures: A Meta-analysis," *Psychoneuroendocrinology* 86 (2017): 152–68, https://doi.org/10.1016/j.psyneuen.2017.08.008.

Chapter 5. Get Organized: Deep Core Training for Asana

1. Henri Cole, "Seamus Heaney: The Art of Poetry No. 75," *Paris Review* 144, 1997, www.theparisreview.org/authors/4028/henri-cole.
2. A small sampling of the many systemic reviews and studies regarding the effects of yoga, meditation, and pranayama on the brain and body shows a slice of the broad consensus: mind-body interventions promote myriad psychoneuroimmunological improvements, including emotional regulation, somatosensory awareness, stress resilience, and learning skills such as concentration and attention. Refer to Clara Snijders, Lotta-Katrin Pries, Noemi Sgammeglia, Nagy A. Youssef, Ghazi Al Jowf, Laurence de Nijs, Sinan Guloksuz, and Bart P. F. Rutten, "Resilience against Traumatic Stress: Current Developments and Future Directions," *Frontiers in Psychiatry* 9 (2018): 676, www.frontiersin.org/articles/10.3389/fpsyt.2018.00676/full; Crystal L. Park, Lucy Finkelstein-Fox, Erik Groessl, A. Rani Elwy, "Exploring How Different Types of Yoga Change Psychological Resources and Emotional Well-Being across a Single Session," *Complementary Therapies in Medicine* 49 (March 2020): 102354, www.ncbi.nlm.nih.gov/pmc/articles/PMC7081324/.

Chapter 6. Stay Centered: Motion Control Training for Asana

1. Alan Watts, *What Is Zen?* (Novato, CA: New World Library, 2010), 53.

Chapter 7. Feel Refreshed: Rest, Reflect, and Regroup

1. Robert H. Gass, "Robert H. Gass Quotes," goodreads, n.d., www.goodreads.com/autho/quotes/21107.Robert_H_Gass.

2. I. K. Taimni, *The Science of Yoga: The Yoga-Sutras of Patanjali in Sanskrit with Transliteration in Roman, Translation and Commentary in English* (Adyar, Chennai, India/Wheaton, IL: Theosophical Publishing House/Quest Books, 1999), Sutras II.3, 4, 5, 6, 7, 8, 9; pp. 130–52.

3. Georg Feuerstein, *The Yoga Tradition: Its History, Literature, Philosophy and Practice* (Chino Valley, AZ: Hohm Press, 2001).

4. Taimni, *Science of Yoga*, Sutra I.3, p. 10.

5. To learn more about the psychoneuroimmunological effects of yoga and other MBIs, consider reading the following books: Bonnie Badenoch, *The Heart of Trauma: Healing the Embodied Brain in the Context of Relationships* (New York: W. W. Norton, 2017); Rick Hanson, with Richard Mendius, *Buddha's Brain: The Practical Neuroscience of Happiness, Love, and Wisdom* (Oakland, CA: New Harbinger Publications, 2009); Jon Kabat-Zinn, *The Healing Power of Mindfulness: A New Way of Being* (New York: Hachette Books, 2018); Bessel A. van der Kolk, *The Body Keeps the Score: Brain, Mind, and Body in the Healing of Trauma* (New York: Penguin Books, 2014).

6. J. M. Kilmer and R. N. Lemon, "What We Know Currently about Mirror Neurons." *Current Biology* 23, no. 23 (2013): R1057–62, https://doi.org/10.1016/j.cub.2013.10.051; Cecilia Heyes and Caroline Catmur, "What Happened to Mirror Neurons?" *Perspectives on Psychological Science* 17, no. 1 (2022): 153–68, https://doi.org/10.1177/1745691621990638.

7. Stephen Porges, *Pocket Guide to Polyvagal Theory: The Transformative Power of Feeling Safe*, Norton Series on Interpersonal Neurobiology (New York: W. W. Norton, 2017), 47.

8. The evolution of body-imaging technology, such as functional magnetic resonance imaging (fMRI), reveals how we respond to stimuli by mapping blood flow and measuring activity in different areas of the brain. When combined with advancements in molecular biology, these brain maps inform an increasingly detailed view into how mind state—that is, arousal—produces endocrine, immune, and nervous system effects. For more information, read Ivana Buric, Miguel Farias, Jonathan Jong, Christopher Mee, and Inti A. Brazil, "What Is the Molecular Signature of Mind–Body Interventions? A Systematic Review of Gene Expression Changes Induced by Meditation and Related Practices," *Frontiers in Immunology* 8 (2017): 670, doi: 10.3389/fimmu.2017.00670.

9. Neha P. Gothe, Imadh Khan, Jessica Hayes, Emily Erlenbach, and Jessica S. Damoiseaux, "Yoga Effects on Brain Health: A Systematic

Review of the Current Literature," *Brain Plasticity* 5, no. 1 (2019): 105–22, https://doi.org/10.3233/BPL-190084.

10. Refer to these articles for more detailed discussion about the psycho-neurology of yoga practice: Acevedo et al., "The Neural Mechanisms of Meditative Practices"; Snijders et al., "Resilience against Traumatic Stress"; and Park et al., "Exploring How Different Types of Yoga Change Psychological Resources."

Chapter 8. Yoga Forward: Go Your Own Way

1. Horace, "Horace Quotes," *BrainyQuote*, 2022, www.brainyquote.com /quotes/horace_382608.

ABOUT THE AUTHOR

Mary Richards, MS, C-IAYT, E-RYT500, YACEP, began practicing yoga in 1992, and teaching in 2002. Her teaching and practice are informed by her deep, abiding interest in and study of anatomy and kinesiology. Mary has completed credited coursework with labs in anatomy, physiology, kinesiology, and biology. Additionally, she holds a master of science in yoga therapy from Maryland University of Integrative Health. She has also completed observation hours at physical therapy facilities specializing in orthopedics and sports medicine. Mary is passionate about sharing her experience in yoga therapeutics and other healing modalities to help others cope with—and ideally, prevent—injury to the joint segments of the body, especially the weight-bearing joints of the lower extremities.

Mary teaches online and in-person workshops. She has presented case studies at research symposia regarding yoga therapeutics, published articles in *Yoga Journal*, and appeared on podcasts. Information about her offerings may be found on her website (www .yogawithmaryrichards.com). When she's not at home or on the mat somewhere, she can be found hugging trees and worshipping dirt at her family's simple yet serviceable cabin in the Blue Ridge Mountains of Rockbridge County, Virginia.

ABOUT THE ILLUSTRATOR

Lili Robins graduated with a bachelor of arts in fine arts from George Washington University and began working in design studios a couple years before graduation. After graduation she polished her news graphics and airbrush skills during a year at the local affiliate of ABC News, then went on to freelance for many Washington, D.C.–area organizations including Time-Life Books, National Geographic Advertising, National Oceanic and Atmospheric Administration, and the Smithsonian Institution (Gems and Mineral Hall, Oceans Planet Exhibit of the Natural History Museum). She later worked in the Virginia public schools teaching high school art, during which time she began a new yoga practice.

Yoga had so much to offer that it inspired Lili to make a big career change. She became a certified yoga teacher, yoga therapist, yoga studio owner, and Yoga Alliance 200-RYT school director in Fredericksburg, Virginia. It was during this decade devoted to yoga that Lili began working regularly with Mary Richards. Soon Mary was incorporated into the teacher training curriculum, and when faced with the COVID regulations, Mary brought her lessons seamlessly to the Zoom platform. Lili served as host, coordinator, and Mary wrangler. It was their work together during the pandemic that led to the illustrations for *Teach People, Not Poses*.